Holograr

5 Keys to Nervous System Consciousness

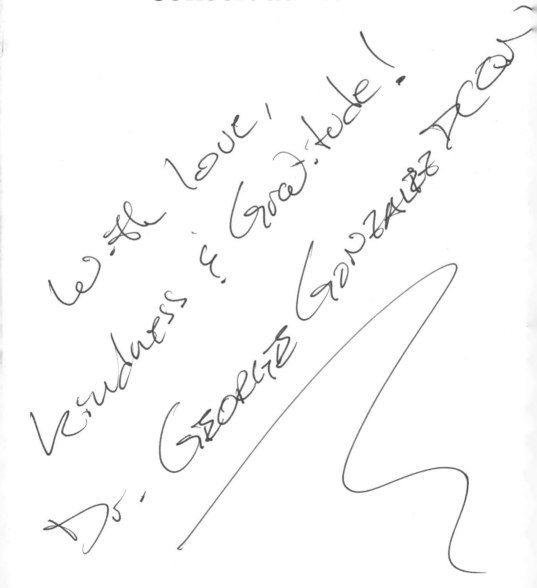

With love!

Kindness & Gratitude!

Dr. George Gonzalez

Holographic Healing

5 Keys to Nervous System Consciousness

George Gonzalez, DC, QN

Book Cover design by Cathi Stevenson
www.bookcoverexpress.com

Book Edited by Heather Marsh
www.classicediting.com

Interior Design by Rudy Milanovich
rudy@wizardvision.com

Soft Cover Book ISBN: 978-0-9855207-0-0
Electronic Book ISBN: 978-0-9855207-1-7

Dedication

I dedicate this book to my family, with the most sincere gratitude. Without them I shudder to think what my life would have been. Through their sacrifice and hard work I've been allowed to shine. Their unconditional love and support have allowed this work to be accomplished.

To…

The loves of my life…my wife Lori and my daughter Gabrielle.

My mother and father, Ludivina and Refugio Gonzalez, for without them none of this would exist.

My brothers, who have been my heroes for as long as I can remember: my oldest brother, Refugio Gonzalez, and his children Luke, Emmanuel, Simeon and Danni; and my older brother, Juan Carlos Gonzalez, and his wife Paola and their children Sabrina, Sebastian, Nico and Sophia.

Lori's parents, Tina and Vicente Guzman, for treating me as their own child.

And special thanks to Lori's brother, whose skills compliment my weaknesses and who has contributed greatly to Quantum Neurology®, Dan Guzman, and his wife Michelle and daughters Alexandria and Olivia.

Acknowledgments

I attribute my skills to hard work and the guidance of my many masters, teachers, family, friends and experiences.

I attribute my gifts to the ability to connect with a consciousness greater than my own understanding. For that reason I would like to thank the Universal Consciousness we share which allows us to have this interaction.

I have so many people to thank it's difficult to get started for fear that I'll forget someone. I would like to thank all the doctors that have dedicated themselves to learning Quantum Neurology® and providing Nervous System rehabilitation services to their patients. I would also like to acknowledge and thank all the recipients of Quantum Neurology Rehabilitation. It is in their need that these concepts have surfaced.

I would like to thank the present and future Quantum Neurologists™ for their contribution to Nervous System exploration. I especially would like to thank Dr. David Pascal, who has followed me for my entire professional career. He was my first student, my first Quantum Neurologist, and he is a close friend and confidant. His use of Quantum Neurology® to enhance elite athletic performance has produced medals and world record times in every major track event the world. I would also like to thank Dr. Elizabeth Hesse Sheehan, who was the first doctor to apply our neurological rehabilitation principles to a patient population affected with Lyme disease, chronic illness and Autism Spectrum Disorder; Dr. James Sheen, in his expansion of Nervous System care and healing principals; and Dr. Chris Cormier, for expanding our understanding of what is possible in the endocrine system and applying these principles to new frontiers.

I would like to acknowledge the special people in my career who supported, housed and fed me and my family—all while encouraging me when I did not believe in myself. These people include Dr. Edward Chauvin and family, Dr. Woody & Mary Beck and family, Dr. Ron & Janet

Stellmacher, Dr. Torry & Lexi Hinson, Dr. Chase Hayden and family, Dr. Andrew & Cathy Tolk and family, and Dr. Tom Weiland and his family.

I would like to thank my special friend Angelo Agon, who invested his time in me when I was a student and taught me many of the healing principles and philosophies contained within this book. His guidance through my training with Dr. Bob and Lisa Curry of Standard Process of Southern California gave me a strong healing philosophy in nutrition, whole foods and real vs. synthetic concepts. When I was a student, Angelo guided me to study with the best natural healing doctors in the world. Although at the time I did not realize it, studying with the best early in my career has fostered the growth and skill that I have today.

To all my teachers, masters and mentors, with special thanks to:

—Dr. Tobi Watkinson for bringing me back from a near fatal mold exposure and teaching me how to trust the Nervous System to guide the patients' care.

—Dr. Bob and Lisa Curry for providing a guiding light for doctors to explore the healing powers of the Nervous System available through food, nutrition and natural healing.

—Dr. Scott Lander for being a friend and a mentor in chiropractic.

—Dr. Michael Dobbins for being a wonderful friend and mentor who has made it his mission to educate doctors on the uses of foods and whole food concentrates to maximize healing.

—Drs. Scott and Deb Walker for their support and the gifts they share with the world through their work of Neuro Emotional Technique®. The healing available through their work is astonishing. Their kindness in teaching and mentorship has made me a better person, doctor and teacher. Thank you.

—Dr. Dick Versendal for teaching me his powerful version of Nervous System guided care.

—Dr. Marc Pick, my first chiropractor, who leads by example and taught me the importance of Nervous System based care by being the first to help Lori after her injury.

—Kyle Morgan, D.O. and A.J. Deeds for developing a system that has allowed my body to heal after 20 years of struggling with my weight.

—Grand Master Gary Lam, through whose training I focused on taking center in my life, health, family and career. His unique and advanced understanding of the Nervous System cultivation and expansion has been a great inspiration to my work.

—Grand Master Nene Gaabucayan for teaching me how to personally develop my Nervous System in ways I never thought possible. His mastery of layering the Nervous System in its development is revolutionary.

—Suzannah Galland for being such a dear friend. Her life and business coaching have saved me from ruin and steered me toward the life of my dreams.

—Marco Aiello for creating the soundtrack of our lives.

—Dr. Steve Hoffman for sharing his gifts and talents. This book was initiated by his presentation on the importance of having a book. This process has made me learn how to define myself in ways I could not have previously. Thank you!

—Dr. Howard and Christine Cohn for being masters of manifesting health, wealth and love. Thank you for sharing and teaching me how to go for it!

—Ed and Mary Miller of Impac Inc. for your support and guidance in this niche industry that we share. Without your help I may have never taken flight.

To my Aikido family—

Seiseki Abe Sensei, Take Shigemichi Sensei, Haruo Matsuoka Sensei, Kinoshita Sensei, Kato Sensei and all my sempai and kohai. My life has a special meaning shaped by the experiences we shared together. Thank you for teaching me the beauty and power available through our Nervous System.

To my closest friends—

The Striegel Brothers—Stephen, Shawn and Scott. I thank you for all the love, laughter and support, especially at my lowest moments.

A special dedication to the families affected by chronic illness, autoimmune and autism spectrum disorder. I am humbled by the drive and focus of these families to find answers to help their loved ones. It is their drive and focus that makes me feel everything will be okay. I would especially like to thank Tami Duncan and Rita Gerald of the LIA Foundation at www.LymeInducedAutism.com, and Dana Gorman from Thriiive.com, for helping educate people about Nervous System rehabilitation and Quantum Neurology®. I would also like to thank the doctors that take on these challenging cases and help families recover their Nervous Systems.

I would especially like to thank Maribel Jimenez, book project coordinator; Heather Marsh, book editor; and Keith Leon, book project coach. It is with their experience and expertise I've been able to write this book and bring this important information to the public in a short period of time. I thank you for your contribution, hard work and dedication.

With love, kindness and gratitude,

George Gonzalez, DC, QN
Doctor of Chiropractic, Quantum Neurologist™
Founder of Quantum Neurology® Rehabilitation
www.QuantumNeurology.com

Introduction

My life's work was revealed to me through the journey of my wife's moderate spinal cord injury and recovery. My wife, Lori, returned home from a massage one day, barely able to walk. A massage therapist had performed a manipulation that severely injured Lori's spine. Pain ran from her lower back and down her legs. She was completely numb below the navel, from her groin and backside, down the back of her legs to the bottoms of her feet. She was barely able to walk because all she could feel was the excruciating pain of her bones as they touched the ground.

I was completing my last trimester of chiropractic school but nothing I had learned in school had prepared me for this. I could not find any doctors of any profession who could tell us what was wrong or suggest any realistic treatment options. Lori's health began to decline quickly, and I was desperate to get her well.

Our first sign of hope came during a session with Marc Pick, DC, who was well versed in neurology. In one session, Dr. Pick was able to get Lori's deep tendon reflexes below the waist to come back. This dramatic shift happened emotionally and physically and woke me up to the amazing healing power within the Nervous System. It was exhilarating to see immediate healing. As a cold, closed plant will open and expand to receive the warmth from the sun's rays, so will our Nervous System, when collapsed in injury, expand into its ability and function. With an exacting evaluation and simple, well-focused corrections, her damaged nerve function was restored. Nothing was added to her body, and nothing was removed. Simply, the stimulation of her Nervous System, in very specific ways, elicited the lost function to return.

At that moment I lost my fear and intimidation of "neurology." My misconceptions of neurology being complicated and difficult had lifted. I immersed myself in study and used my background in martial arts to expand my thinking.

Using my wife's Nervous System as our guide, I developed a functional evaluation of the Nervous System. I found a way to organize and sequence traditional neurology testing principles within a *healing form*. These principles are the gold standard of neurology testing, taught to every doctor in the world.

The healing form is my strategic evaluation of these principles. Similar to martial arts, the healing form is practiced in a particular sequence. This ensures proper and consistent evaluation of the entire Nervous System from patient to patient. Each person has a unique pattern of weaknesses that becomes evident throughout the evaluation. This consistency allows each person to have a unique experience, with a customized rehabilitation to complement his or her Nervous System and goals.

After many years of using our standardized neurological evaluation, my students and I have gleaned information about the Nervous System. My wife's rehabilitation led us to new discoveries of how the Nervous System maps out. We have learned how to better describe and evaluate the Nervous System. We have discovered that the Nervous System extends beyond what we were taught in school—that the Nervous System is simply the brain, spinal cord and nerves. We now understand that the Nervous System includes every action and communication available to the body. It includes the physical body and all aspects of the nonphysical body, also known as the energetic body, bioenergetic field, aura or LightBody. It includes the mind, thoughts, emotions and spiritual connections.

We consistently see immediate neurological change when applying these principles to the Nervous System. Everything we've been taught about the Nervous System is outdated—as outdated as the solar system model only having nine planets taught when I was in school. I'm not saying that neurology training in place is not accurate. I'm simply stating that I have discovered a new vantage point from which we can explore the Nervous System. We can now explore and recover the Nervous System through its functions and abilities. We correct the body through range of motion and during its action. We now have a command of the Nervous System as the electrician commands the flow of a home's electricity through the breaker box and its wires.

Our modern understanding of the Nervous System must reach beyond the five senses. It must reflect the multiple layers of communication that occur within our Nervous System and the most advanced principles of quantum physics. It must allow for instantaneous and constant communications throughout the body and the universe. Ultimately we do not know what the answers are. We can only use models to help us understand and wrap our minds around the complexity of our *Holographic Nervous System.*

Holographic communication can be described as the *software of the Nervous System.* Holographs allow us to describe the multiple layers of communications that occur simultaneously. They are further characterized by the fact that all information of the Nervous System is contained within its smallest unit: a single cell.

Most people recognize a holograph as a three-dimensional image created with laser beams reflecting off an object. The holographic image can be viewed from different perspectives as if it were sitting on the table in front of you. If you take the holographic image and cut it into four pieces, you will not have the four corners of the original image. You will actually have four, identical three-dimensional images. If you continue to tear these pieces again, each of the pieces will contain the entire image, no matter how small you managed to tear them.

The body fits into the holographic model because all the information is contained within its smallest unit. Every cell contains genetic material we recognize to be DNA, which can be transferred and cloned, creating an entire new self. The holographic model applied to the Nervous System allows for the instantaneous communication that occurs throughout the body and the universe.

Expanding on the concept discovered by Fritz-Albert Popp, PhD, that each cell communicates through emissions of light called biophotons, the biophoton of light is also known to carry intelligence. This intelligent biophoton communication occurs throughout the body and at the speed of light.

In this book I present my theory of how the physical body generates the life we experience. I propose that the emission of light from each individual cell, when considered in its totality—trillions and trillions of cells—generates a light force, a biophotonic field, that is responsible for our body's integration and communication. This light force is the nonphysical communication system within our physical frame. I call this phenomenon the *LightBody*. The intellectual mind is not in the brain. The mind cannot be isolated to a single location within the brain or the Nervous System. Large computer systems that can measure or visualize thought processes are not locating a thought. They simply visualize the part of the Brain or Nerve Tissue that is active when that thought occurs.

I believe the LightBody contains all of our nonphysical attributes, including our mind, thoughts, emotions and capacity for love, joy and spiritual connection. The Big Idea is that the LightBody seems to be the nonphysical projected holograph of the self. The LightBody is responsible for the connection and communication between us and everything in our universe.

Using this concept of the LightBody, my students and I have discovered new methods of cultivating and expanding the Nervous System. It has been our experience that when the Nervous System is expanded it will heal itself. We have found that light therapy bridges the communication within the Nervous System. Where there is no communication, there are disease and dysfunction.

The idea is simple: we want to maximize the body's ability to communicate and perform actions. We do this by evaluating the Nervous System and using light therapy as a stimulus for the rehabilitation of lost function.

When we used these concepts, we began to see immediate improvement in Lori's recovery, and I started seeing these results with my other patients.

I saw pain go away immediately, range of motion return and function restored. Although I did not realize it at the time, I was well on my way to developing what is now known as Quantum Neurology® Rehabilitation.

This work has transformed my life. Quantum Neurology® has delivered amazing healing and world record performances. In my wife's case, her complete recovery from sensory paralysis and giving birth to our child is, by far, the sweetest personal victory. Quantum Neurology rehabilitation is healing the world. Doctors from around the world learn these methods though hands-on seminars, home and online training. To find a Quantum Neurology® trained practitioner near you, and learn more about Neurological Rehabilitation and Holographic Healing, visit our website at www.QuantumNeurology.com.

This work has been a blessing in my life, and I truly hope that it will be one in yours.

With Love, Kindness & Gratitude,

George Gonzalez, DC, QN
Doctor of Chiropractic, Quantum Neurologist™
Founder of Quantum Neurology® Rehabilitation

"The doctor of the future will give no medicine, but will interest his patients in the care of the human frame, in diet, and in the cause and prevention of disease."

—Thomas Edison, Inventor

Table of Contents

Chapter 1

HOLOGRAPHIC HEALING

Welcome to the Hologram!

Holographic Healing… What does that mean?

Healing, of course, we recognize as a natural process that our body goes through to recover from infection, injury, illness or a condition.

Yes, but what does holographic mean? And how does it relate to healing?

Holographic refers to a concept that all information is contained within the smallest unit. A seed contains all the information of a tree. A fertilized embryo contains all the genetic information of both parents. As the embryo grows to adulthood, every cell carries and contributes to the ongoing genetic record. Our genetic code is a record of everything that is perceived and experienced by our Nervous System. This record contains every aspect of our life's experiences, mental, emotional and spiritual states, as well as health, physical conditions, injuries and infections, and how they were overcome. It records every aspect of who we are, as it has for all our ancestors, since the dawn of time.

In nature, we often see the holographic concept exhibited. Insects and animals can function individually, but in a group dynamic the group exhibits its own lifelike characteristics. Great examples of this are: bees in their swarms, birds in their flock formations, schools of fish and their reactivity to movement, dogs acting strangely before earthquakes, animals running toward high ground before a tsunami tidal wave. This concept is also recognized in humans as our ability to move without bumping into each other. Whether we are walking or driving in a crowded area, we seem to avoid hitting each other most of the time. We all seem to have this awareness, a knowing, a connection to everything and everyone around us. We know when we are being stared at. We think of someone and then they call. These are all examples of holographic communication. The holographic concept is interesting because the information and communication we are describing does not exist physically. We cannot pinpoint or locate the tree in the seed, or the human in the DNA, but we know it's there because that's where everything comes from. Somehow the genetic material we call DNA records all the information of our lives and stores, unscrambles and then uses it in a way we know very little about. We refer to this type of information processing and the ability to access it instantaneously throughout our life as holographic. It can simply be described as the *software of our Nervous System.*

Holographic healing allows us to heal our minds and bodies by using the concepts of the holographic model. I'm sure this may seem far-fetched and abstract. My intention is to connect the dots in such a way that you recognize you are the center of your universe. Your Nervous System generates your reality experience from moment to moment. Most importantly, I would like you to grasp the POWERFUL HEALING available within your Nervous System and how to access it!

The Nervous System

"A rainbow is a holographic projection of light through water.
Life is a holographic projection of light through our Nervous System."
— George Gonzalez, DC, QN

In order to understand holographic healing, we must first understand the instrument we call our body.

I refer to the body as the Nervous System because it is more descriptive of what we are as beings. The concept of our Nervous System represents everything we are. It includes everything we know and everything we do not know about ourselves. It includes all recognized and unrecognized communications and actions available through our body.

It includes the physical body, the bioenergetic field, the aura, the Holographic LightBody and any other existence or communication associated with the body that has not yet been discovered.

Life is the *experience of living*. The Nervous System is the platform on which *Life* is played. It carries our consciousness and our intellectual mind and generates the experience we are having. It controls our physical body and our movements. It allocates resources for managing all the tasks within the body. It provides access to the external environment which we experience with our five senses: seeing, hearing, smelling, tasting and touching. It also provides access to our nonphysical experience: our mind, thoughts, emotions and spiritual connections.

We appreciate health especially when we deal with injury or illness. What is difficult to understand is: What is health? What generates health in our bodies? Why is there so much conflicting information about how to achieve and maintain health?

I've worked with many highly qualified doctors. When I mention to them the importance of Nervous System health, they all agree in unison. Remarks such as "well, of course the Nervous System controls everything" are a common response. Although this may be a common understanding among the doctors of the world, this is not understood by the public at large. This book informs the public of advanced healing principles used successfully by elite doctors around the world.

In school, doctors are taught that the Nervous System is comprised of the brain, spinal cord and nerves. Doctors are taught that the brain controls the entire body and the mind is located somewhere inside the head. In actuality, the Nervous System is much more intricate than we were originally taught. Each nerve that exits the spine can be thought of as a wire that connects four main areas of the body. Each nerve wire will connect to specific muscles, tissues, organs and bones. Just as the leaves of a plant depend on a branch to supply them with life-sustaining resources, the quality of communication available within the nerve wire is directly related to the health of our muscles, tissues, organs and bones. Each of these areas can be individually damaged. Damaged or weak areas will pull energy from stronger areas sharing the same nerve wire. Eventually, individually damaged areas can contribute to the overall weakness of everything along that nerve wire. A damaged nerve wire can contribute to the overall weaknesses and eventual collapse of the Nervous System.

Our Nervous System is the primary indicator of our health. When we understand how the Nervous System works and how it's integrated into the universe, we can understand how to evaluate and strengthen our connection with the body, mind, surroundings and with others to experience happier and more fulfilling lives.

Trial by Fire

I did not understand holographic healing as I developed Quantum Neurology®. This information has revealed itself through my years of clinical experience, teaching and consulting in Nervous System rehabilitation. There are moments in life we have to trust the Nervous System. In situations where we don't have all the answers, or the luxury of time, we have to trust the Nervous System. Most would call this *listening to our gut (or physical) instinct*. Others refer to the ability to focus and act without thought as being "in the zone." This is when you let your Nervous System do its job without "you" getting in the way.

I was traveling through the San Francisco bay area when I received one of those life-changing calls. My close friend Dr. Edward Chauvin was in an intensive care unit in Louisiana with a severe aneurysm. I returned home to Los Angeles and kept in close contact with Edward's family. He went into surgery the next day guided by his college roommate, Dr. Julian Bailes, a neurosurgeon who developed the procedure to correct the aneurysm Edward had suffered. There are no coincidences in my world, and I made plans to be in Louisiana as quickly as possible.

We are so fortunate and grateful that Edward survived the emergency surgery. When I arrived in Louisiana four days after his surgery, Edward's son Ben picked me up from the airport. During the two hour drive, he told me that the doctors recommended around-the-clock care for at least one year. Their family had decided to fire his office staff and was questioning what to do with his practice and who they would hire to care for Edward.

Ben and I were greeted at the hospital by Edward's youngest son, Patrick. When I first saw Edward in the intensive care unit, he had a stroke-like paralysis pattern. He was paralyzed on the left side of his body and the right side of his face. He was barely conscious and fading in and out. His speech was slurred and difficult to comprehend. There was a tube draining the fluid from his head and the typical IV and chest monitoring equipment. I only had five minutes with him, so I had to focus on strengthening the most important nerves, those primarily responsible for his body's ability to rest, digest and heal itself.

The nurses and doctors looked over inquisitively but were not interested enough to come and watch. There's definitely curiosity when an untrained person watches me conduct a neurological rehabilitation for the first time. After all, I was using a flashing red light over Edward's head and scar, while having him say: Nyuck, Nyuck, Nyuck, Nyuck. Kuh, Kuh, Kuh, Kuh. Juh, Juh, Juh, Juh. I was asking him to activate Cranial Nerve X (ten) which controls the specific muscles associated with recovering speech and swallowing. The same nerve that allows us to make those sounds contributes to our ability to maintain blood pressure, respiration rate, activate digestion and detoxification and countless other things associated to resting, digesting and healing. My experience has been that strengthening the muscles available on that nerve wire will stimulate and strengthen the body's ability to heal itself. After my focused corrections, I prayed with the family and left Edward to heal.

The next day, Ben and I arrived at the ICU to find out that Edward had responded so well the evening prior he had been transferred into his own room. To our delight and amazement, he was speaking clearly and moving both arms, both legs and his face was symmetrical. Gone were all signs of paralysis in his face or body. The drainage tube had been removed from his head. He was extremely exhausted yet more coherent than the last time we spoke. His leaving the ICU was a celebrated victory that inspired us and gave us hope. I immediately focused on continuing to reintegrate his Nervous System using the same principles and techniques I discovered while rehabilitating my wife through her injury. I worked on him for two short sessions that day, once in the morning and once in the evening. During that time, I evaluated and strengthened every major nerve in his body. As he rested, we waited to see how his body responded to rehabilitation.

Watching Edward wake up after two days of sleeping was a welcome relief. He simply opened his eyes and sat up. He was physically exhausted and needed to recover his strength, yet from that moment on his Nervous System was back online, and he was physically and mentally integrated and able to communicate. Eleven days after his surgery, he walked out of the hospital with *zero* neurological deficits. He returned to work 29 days after surgery and has been practicing full-time since.

It was truly amazing to watch the light come back into Edward's face while we were making neurological corrections. With each correction, his strength, energy and sense of humor improved. It was through this experience that I realized the Nervous System is far greater than we were ever taught or could even imagine. I had witnessed a severely disabled man restored in a matter of days. He is a medical miracle.

Nervous System Software: Holograph Version 1.0

Let's get back to the concept of the hologram.

What hologram?

The one you are living in.

You are living a holographic experience.

Don't worry. It's OK to be asking yourself, "What is this guy talking about?" It will all begin making sense once you understand the Nervous System and how it communicates.

I'm sure you would agree that you have intelligence and that you are conscious. Have you ever wondered where in the brain or body that intelligence and consciousness exist? Most people believe it's located somewhere between our ears. After all, there is an abundance of Nervous

System tissue we call the brain located within the skull. Various machines which measure Nervous System activity have been cross-referenced with mental function. But no machine can locate and isolate intelligence or consciousness within the physical body. Machines simply visualize which part of the Nervous System is active while a thought occurs.

A simple polygraph, commonly known as a lie detector machine, uses various *autonomic* (automatic nervous system) responses to measure the effect a thought has on the body. Autonomic responses measured by these types of machines include heart rate, blood pressure, galvanic skin response, respiratory rate, body temperature and pupil reactivity, to name a few. Notice the need to measure various parts of the body and not simply the head. This is because each thought has an effect on the entire body. I'm confident you have experienced an emotional flush as a result of a thought. Hearing bad news can send a chill down your spine. When you are delighted, your entire body gets a sudden surge of joy. Thoughts and emotions are not head-only experiences; they are Nervous System experiences.

Where Does Intelligent Consciousness Exist?

I am proposing that your intelligent consciousness is not physical. The physical body and nerve tissue are the hardware and hard wires of the Nervous System. Your nonphysical self—your mind, thoughts, emotions and spiritual connections—is the software of the Nervous System. Similarly, as your experience on a computer or the Internet cannot be located to a single spot on the computer hardware, your body is simply the physical interface of the Nervous System. The nonphysical experience we know as *Life* cannot be isolated to a single spot within the body.

The concept of the nonphysical self can be overwhelming. We are so used to thinking of our physical existence that it can be difficult to comprehend the nonphysical. We've been taught to ignore experience and intuition and only rely on things which are measured through our five senses (sight, hearing, smell, taste and touch). I'm sure you see the dilemma: we cannot physically measure the nonphysical, so we have difficulty quantifying its existence outside of our personal experiences.

Our Nervous System has the incredible ability to maintain constant and instantaneous communication with trillions of cells, multiple life-sustaining systems and activities, mental functions, self communications, interpersonal communications and maintain our spiritual connections. Your nonphysical self is not limited by space, time or location. In an instant you can be transported onto a relaxing beach, sand sticking to your back, warm sun against your skin, surrounded by the sounds of waves, birds and children playing nearby. As you bask in that moment, where are you? What allows you to experience the beach when you are not physically there? These and many other manifestations of your nonphysical self can be described as holographic.

Looking at the body and Nervous System in this way allows us to explore possibilities unavailable through the five senses and physical reality. It opens us up to a full understanding of the Nervous System and not just to what can be measured.

The concept of describing life's experience as holographic is not new, although my phrasing and explanation of it may be unique. Many cultural traditions explain concepts through holographic models.

Many people are familiar with the concept of a voodoo doll, in which a practitioner attaches physical samples, such as hair or personal items belonging to a person, to a doll. The doll becomes a holographic representation of the victim. Poking the doll with needles is said to cause pain to the same location on the victim's body. The victim can be affected anywhere in the world and, in theory, anywhere in the universe because this intention works in the realm of the nonphysical, and is beyond time and space.

Prayer and spiritual services are another example. A prayer can be described as a good intention or good thought. I believe these good thoughts reach the people for whom they are intended instantly, the moment they are created.

Focused healing through prayer or meditation can be done while in the physical presence of the person, or from a great distance. Directing healing intention from a distance is called remote healing. All of these ideas can ultimately be described as holographic communications. Understanding these concepts can give us a sense of empowerment and amazement at what is truly possible through our Nervous System.

The Nervous System is such an amazing instrument, capable of extremely intricate inter-dimensional communication—and we each have this amazing intelligence within us. This intelligence logistically co-ordinates every function of our chaotic lives, from attending meetings, remembering names and participating in events, down to the locations, purposes and actions of every cell in our bodies. This same intelligence can be focused toward rebuilding, healing and expanding the Nervous System. It has been my experience that—when the Nervous System is focused on healing and strengthening—the body will heal itself.

Chapter 2

THE GIFT

Life was challenging, yet promising, for my wife and me in our late 20s, as with any couple with a spouse going through doctorate training. I was in my last term of chiropractic school before graduation. My young wife, Lori, was beautiful, healthy, physically active and working as an administrative assistant. We had planned our lives. I was looking for an office to do my internship. And once we settled in an office, we wanted to have children. We did not foresee any obstacles. We soon learned that the obstacles in life could change our plans in one moment.

The stress of supporting me through school was taking a toll on Lori. At the advice of some friends, I decided to treat her to a massage. Lori was always very cautious about having body work done. She had a stable broken vertebra in her low back at the level of L5. This vertebra is commonly broken in teenage girls who do gymnastics and ride horses. Lori told the massage therapist about her back condition and specifically asked that no work be done on her lower back. The masseuse, against Lori's wishes, and against her licensure, manipulated Lori's lower spine by a performing a downward thrust. Lori immediately felt a mild itching sensation on the bottoms of her feet.

By that evening, Lori was experiencing severe pain in her low back, legs and feet. In fact, all the areas that would touch a saddle if she were riding a horse were completely numb: her groin, backside, the back of her legs, and the bottoms of her feet. Without the sensation on the bottoms of her feet, walking was very painful and difficult. She described it as similar to walking barefoot on sharp rocks as she could feel the bones and ligaments but not the flesh of her feet.

Lori developed urinary frequency, urgency and incontinence. She could not find a comfortable position sitting, standing or lying down. Warm temperatures and warm water, especially hot baths, exacerbated her symptoms. She could not wear high heels or shoes that fully covered her feet.

What I did not fully understand at that time was that her Nervous System had been damaged, and these patterns of loss and symptoms were the breakdown of communication within her Nervous System. After a tiring and unsuccessful search for doctors and a treatment that could help her, Lori finally experienced a breakthrough in a session with Dr. Marc Pick. He is a world renowned Doctor of Chiropractic who lectures on Sacral Occipital Technique (SOT) and clinical neurology. Using his system of analysis, he extensively mapped out Lori's Nervous System.

That one, incredible day, I sat with Lori during her first exam by Dr. Pick. With each neurological evaluation, I sank deeper in terror as she failed the functional tests, which indicated possible permanent nerve damage. Initially, these functional tests were just answers to exam questions. The horror was that they might define the new boundaries of my wife's Nervous System. Most people experience the simple knee-jerk response activated when our legs are dangling and one leg is tapped just below the kneecap. Lori had lost that and all other reflexes below the waist. She was completely numb and unable to feel a pin stick on the saddle areas and bottoms of her feet. She had no plantar response, which means that jabbing and dragging a pointed metal instrument on the bottom of her foot showed no response. Most people would have pulled their entire leg and foot away from that stimulus. Considering the damage she experienced, we were thankful her muscles were still working and had not become weak or atrophied during our search for answers.

So, during that first exam with Dr. Pick, as each demonstration revealed more nerve damage, it took all I had to stay focused and pay attention. That hour, as he measured the parameters of her Nervous System, was one of the most intense hours of my life. The reality of the damage was overwhelming. I was checking out mentally. My mind raced with thoughts of how this would affect our lives. How would we be able to have children? How could I afford the care she deserved? How would I know what she needed? Thoughts of Lori having to live with this damage for the rest of her life were depressing and overwhelming.

My mind was so overwhelmed with the severity of her injury that I barely paid attention to the corrections Dr. Pick performed on Lori. Some stretches on one leg, then he pulled on some of her fingers. The next thing I knew, she was able to pull her leg and foot away from him when he jabbed the bottom of her foot. Watching this and her knee jerk response restored in one session was remarkable. Everything happened so fast that it wasn't until the drive home from the doctor's office that I began to process what had just happened. I pulled over to the side of the road, and all I could do was sit and cry. My excitement was only contained by my understanding of the severity of the damage remaining and fear of the unknown.

It's hard to explain the range of emotions we experienced when Dr. Pick's extensive neurological evaluation unveiled the extent of Lori's damage. The amazing experience of watching her body see instant benefit from Nervous System rehabilitation was the first sign of hope we had toward her healing. This experience led me toward a new direction, one which, over time, has become clear and well-defined. I felt that my life purpose became to research, practice and teach Nervous System cultivation and expansion.

Dr. Pick's single session with Lori initiated her healing. He also gave me the understanding that Nervous System capability dictates quality of life. From that day forward, I dedicated myself to researching neurology while rehabilitating my wife from her moderate spinal cord injury.

Early on, as I developed the rehabilitation techniques, results were slow to appear. I had to perform multiple corrections every day because Lori's Nervous System was so weak. She would re-injure and lose some of her corrections simply by rolling over on the treatment table. Lori's rehabilitation took years and was both emotionally draining and healing, yet it caused me to look for ways to heal that were beyond my intellect and my natural instincts.

The Great Healing Distraction

There is an unwritten rule among health care professionals that caution should be taken when treating family members, because they can become your most difficult patients. There are many facets to this unwritten rule, but the main goal is to protect the doctor and maintain the close relationships that exist with loved ones. In our case, the mental and emotional stress of bearing the responsibility for Lori's care was nearly paralyzing.

During the first few months of her injury, my anger, regret and shame over the circumstances were all-consuming. Lori was struggling to cope with the new challenges of her condition and get through her day. We misdirected our focus and our energy in the hope for an easy solution to return what we felt was stolen from us. We were angry and dissatisfied with the direction our lives had turned, and we began fighting with the massage therapist who injured Lori, and with each other.

Our energy literally became occupied, even locked up at times, with the negative emotions and thought patterns. For example, when we fell into a mental fantasy of vindication and payback, we noticed that it created an emotional rush, a surge of false empowerment in the delusion of the fantasy.

I found it difficult to function carrying all these emotions. I couldn't sleep, I gained weight, and I experienced pain even though my body was not injured. I discussed these emotions with Lori, who was struggling, too. We came to a profound conclusion: she would never heal if we kept wasting our energy on things that did not contribute to her healing.

As our delusions of revenge occupied our thought space and blocked the loving energy needed for Lori's healing, I realized this was a recurring phenomenon. It became clear that negative thoughts block the body's ability to heal.

When you indulge in those moments of mental fantasy, I ask you to listen to your Nervous System. What are you feeling? Adrenaline rush? Blood pressure rise? Anxiety? Aggression and depression? Although these negative thoughts may pay dividends in fantasy, they're wasting your energy! Your focus and energy are valuable resources that can be directed toward your body's ability to heal itself.

Would you yell at the captain of a boat for not providing life vests when someone you love is drowning? Or would you instead invest all your energy in saving your loved one? The more severe the health crisis you are in, the more real this becomes.

We were managing Lori's health and at the end of our rope energetically. Our lives were so overwhelmed with managing Lori's care that it became exceedingly obvious that every unsupportive thought cost us energy. This was difficult to notice when we had energy to spare. But when we had reached the limits of our energy threshold, it was as clear as day.

Forgiveness and Healing

Once we realized that holding on to our anger and resentment was a major obstacle in Lori's healing, we had to let it go. Now, that may sound easy, but it was a long and difficult process. We began this process together in prayer, asking for guidance greater than ourselves. We systematically asked for our energy back. We visualized the energetic connections between ourselves and each of the people in our lives, whether living or deceased. We focused on forgiving those who had harmed us and asked for forgiveness from those we had harmed. In that moment, we chose to let go of the certainty of blame and of being victimized, and we exchanged it for the uncertainty of Lori's healing.

I don't like the saying *forgive and forget*. It implies that forgiveness is only attained if you can forget the offense. For me, this implies that you were never wronged or damaged. I feel it's more realistic for someone to learn from experiences and build appropriate boundaries. I'd much rather say *forgive and heal*—a much more realistic indication of what happens when we forgive.

From the moment we changed our focus from fighting those who hurt us, to supporting Lori's healing, we saw immediate improvements. Her gains and corrections lasted longer. She made progress against the constant re-injury of her Nervous System.

I would like to emphasize this was not easy. All my instincts told me to fight, fight, fight. I constantly had to remind myself that fighting wouldn't help. To shift my thinking, I asked myself how each line of thinking contributed to getting what I wanted. Lori was drowning, and I was distracted from saving her by my reactive emotions of anger, resentment, revenge and hate. Forgiveness, for me, had very little to do with creating a fruitful relationship with the person who had hurt my wife. Instead, I invested in taking my energy back from those who had harmed her, and then used that energy to manifest healing.

Although her rehabilitation was slow the first few years, she has made a complete recovery and has regained full sensation in all areas affected by the injury. She no longer suffers from pain in her lower back, legs, or feet. The urinary frequency, urgency, and incontinence issues were resolved. Two to three times per year she may experience an occasional flare up of symptoms, but they last a couple of days until rehabilitation restores her to full health once again.

Residual effects from her injury include not being able to sit in a hardback chair at 90 degrees; she prefers to be more reclined. She can now walk at a brisk pace, but she cannot walk as fast as she could before her injury. She depends on the support of pillows under and between her knees when sleeping to take the stress off her back. In spite of the limitations, she now lives an active lifestyle. And today Lori and I have a beautiful baby girl.

Now, both Lori and I look upon this entire experience as a gift. Lori's case provided the opportunity to fully explore the Nervous System and learn how to measure its effects and boundaries. By seeking to understand the Nervous System, and letting our understanding guide Lori's care, we were able to make decisions about her health and healing without having to rely on doctors' trials and errors, studies, research and the overabundance of information that exists. Instead, we made decisions based on how her body responded to rehabilitation.

In the process of healing Lori's body, we discovered that ultimately we are all in control of our own health, and that our own Nervous System dictates the quality of our lives. We learned to use the Nervous System's ability to guide our care. It allows us to live happier and more fruitful lives to enjoy and share with our family, friends and loved ones.

My experience is an example of what is possible with forgiveness. Focusing on the healing, and letting go of the anger over how Lori was injured, allowed many wonderful gifts to come into our lives. We simply shifted our focus from anger and vengeance to healing. We are not thanking the person who injured Lori, yet we are grateful for the insights and abilities to have made the best of the situation. Lori's rehabilitation guided this work into existence. Countless people have benefited from the concepts of Nervous System rehabilitation, and a new science of Nervous System exploration has emerged.

> *"The most beautiful thing we can experience is the mysterious.*
> *It is the source of all true art and science."*
> —Albert Einstein, Theoretical Physicist

Chapter 3

KEY #1: THE NERVOUS SYSTEM IS CONSCIOUS

The first key to Nervous System Consciousness is the understanding that the source of all healing exists within our bodies. This is referred to in healing circles as *Innate Intelligence* or *Consciousness* and recognized throughout the world in many healing traditions. Each describes their version of the energy that gives us life. Each language has a different name for the intelligence, but to my understanding all refer to the same concept. The Chinese call this energy *Qi* (pronounced "*chi*"), the Japanese call it *Ki* (pronounced "*key*"), and in the East Indian traditions it is called *Prana*. In various religious traditions, this energy is depicted as a glow around a person or a halo around the head.

Every culture seems to have a tradition and understanding of this life force within us. Unfortunately, modern traditions ignore what cannot be measured through the five senses. In my opinion, this has clouded our understanding of the Nervous System and its true capabilities.

We have all heard the adage that we are only using ten percent of the brain. I disagree with this concept because we use our entire Nervous System for every thought and every action. I don't know where this statistic came from, but I guarantee it resulted from the absence of a machine's ability to measure the brain's and Nervous System's capabilities. Our true capabilities are discovered daily. With today's technology, we can learn at incredible speeds. At no other time in history has nearly every person had access to so much information in the world. The increase in technology and new virtual connectivity has been amazing, but connectivity to physical reality has been sacrificed.

In this chapter, I will share how your Nervous System is the center of what gives you life and is the only true indicator of your health. Understanding your Nervous System and its connection to the universe allows you to navigate through life with more direction and purpose, just as understanding the movement of the stars allows you to navigate the globe.

I. Your Nervous System

Learning how to live a Nervous System Conscious *Life* starts with understanding what is at the center of what gives us life and generates our life experience? The answers are found within our Nervous System.

Your Nervous System is much more than what you were taught in school. Your brain and spinal cord are called the *central nervous system*. The nerves which branch off the brain and spinal cord are called *peripheral nerves*. These nerves connect the brain and spinal cord to the rest of the body.

I feel the traditional definition of the Nervous System falls short of explaining its true capabilities when it merely describes the physical hard wiring of the body. The Nervous System actually includes the physical body, energetic body, holographic LightBody and the interactive ability to communicate with different environments: internal, external and nonphysical. The Nervous System is a physical and nonphysical communication interface. The physical communication is experienced through our five senses. The nonphysical Nervous System communication is described as holographic.

Your Nervous System's ability to make intelligent connections to its surroundings exhibits consciousness. These connections allow the Nervous System to make crucial decisions regarding your survival without consulting you. Your body has the ability to instantaneously adjust and react to changes in temperature, blood sugar levels, pH balance, blood pressure, and heart and respiration rates all without your mental contribution. This is evidence of your Nervous System consciousness beyond your mental intellect.

II. Indicators of Health

In quantum physics, to be considered an accurate measurement, the observer's perspective must be included. You may not be the center of the physical Universe, but you are the observer, which makes you the center of *your* universe. Your Nervous System must be included in any measurement for it to be accurate. This simple shift in perspective allows us to use the Nervous System to guide our care. When you do this, you allow your observation to guide your reality. This gives you the ability to hone in on the qualities you desire in life.

Our quality of life is directly related to the connection of our Nervous System with its surroundings. Full disconnection from the space surrounding the body—is death. More integrated connection with our surroundings, is *Life*. When we use the Nervous System as an indicator to guide us in our health and healing, we are using the center point of the universe that generates our experience.

Let's evaluate how our Nervous System connects to the universe using vision as the example. Let's look at its ranges of function (connection), particularly with peripheral vision and central vision. Peripheral vision is our ability to see to our sides while maintaining a focal point. If we put our arms straight out to our sides and look at a point in front of us, then wiggle our fingers, we can bring our hands closer and closer in front of us. Our peripheral vision is how far out to the sides we can see our fingers wiggling. The range in all directions above us and below us is our peripheral vision.

Central vision, or visual acuity, is most recognized as that which is measured by a 20/20 eye chart. It measures how far into the distance we can see and focus. When people damage their vision their visual acuity collapses. Tunnel vision, or losing your range of peripheral vision, is a common sign of vision collapse. When it becomes even more compromised, it can become binocular vision. Binocular vision looks like the two holes that are visualized when looking through binoculars. When a person loses even more visual field, vision is reduced to pinpoints, as if he or she is looking through straws. When visual communication is completely disconnected from the physical universe, blindness occurs. The new reality experience is formed from the remaining senses.

The most important indicator of health is the understanding of how the Nervous System connects to the Universe. If you die, where does the universe go? Where does your experience of this universe go? The universe will exist without your continued contribution, but when your connection to it disappears it causes physical death. With that in mind, by making our connection to the Universe stronger, it gives us a deeper and more integrated *Life* experience!

I am exploring the rules of the universe simply by saying, "Hey, we are multi-dimensional beings. Clean food, air and water nourish and support the body; synthetic chemicals destroy and disconnect the body's ability to interact within the universe." Most people don't think about themselves in this way. They don't realize their body is a communication system or that they can enhance their lives by improving their Nervous System's ability to communicate.

You can make your Nervous System stronger in any area you focus your attention. Your Nervous System generates your *Life* experience.

III. Communication Interface

Our communication interface is how our Nervous System is integrated, or plugged in, to the universe. The Nervous System is a magnificent collection of experience ranges that make up our communication interface. This interface is so intricate that it can manage all of our communication needs. It allows us to communicate with ourselves and each other while managing constant communication within every cell of the body. It receives constant information from the surrounding universe.

We have all seen examples of finely run systems. From businesses to athletics, a group of people who work together in a coordinated effort is amazing. Those who command these skills are often rewarded exponentially beyond other professionals in the same field.

We all know the challenges of working with others. We've all coordinated schedules, missed appointments and have pushed projects back due to minor obstacles. Now consider what is necessary to manage the coordinated effort of trillions and trillions of people. It's mind boggling when you think of the coordinated communication necessary to accomplish anything as a whole. Our Nervous System accomplishes this with our trillions of cells every moment.

Our communication interface—and how we personally integrate with the universe—is a unique experience. Most of us have the ability to see the colors of the visual spectrum (red, orange, yellow, green, blue, indigo and violet). The borders of the visual spectrum, however, are not visible. On the red side of the spectrum, is infrared, which is not visible to the naked human eye. On the violet side of the spectrum, is Ultra Violet (UV), which is also invisible to the naked human eye. This color experience is not the same from person to person. Certain animals and some people can see "colors" in the invisible ranges of infrared and UV. There is no specific marker to indicate that I experience the same light reception ability as everyone else. Anyone may have a bit more or a bit less color range into the ultraviolet or the infrared spectrum.

This would explain how some can see auras, beings and entities that are not visible by others. Animals such as owls have vision in the infrared field. They can track the heat signature of their prey in the darkness of night with their infrared vision. Our Nervous System can receive visual information in a narrow portion of the electromagnetic spectrum. Other non-visible wavelengths on the same electromagnetic spectrum include x-rays, gamma rays, radio waves and microwaves. We know that these waves exist even though we cannot experience them with our five senses.

It is easy to think that we can only have experiences through our five senses, even though we understand the concept that there are things beyond our five senses. Our Nervous System is this interface of experience ranges. We experience light and vibration in very specific ranges.

We experience weight, gravity and the body's ability to hydrate and manage its temperature in very specific ranges. We experience these ranges with our Nervous System, our communication interface.

IV. Nervous System Guided Care

The prevalent attitude of many traditional physicians can be summarized by the following phrases: "I am the doctor. I am smarter, and I know better than you. I, the doctor, decide what is best for you, the patient. If you don't do as I say, you're going to die." These thought forms, perceptions, often provide a very negative experience. It can be described as a *health scare* when the patient is scared into a line of procedures or synthetic medications.

I am suggesting an alternative approach to selecting care for you and your family. My ultimate goal is to show how the Nervous System guides and delivers care that expands and heals the body.

Whether they are meeting a patient for the first time, or care is ongoing, I train doctors in the importance of supportive thought forms when delivering care to patients. In this new way of thinking, the Nervous System's intelligence guides the body to heal itself. The doctor is the coach directing the awareness of the Nervous System to expand its abilities. As Quantum Neurologists, we stimulate the Nervous System's natural healing processes and rehabilitate the actions that cultivate and expand a person's capabilities. Our experience is that, when the Nervous System expands, the body has the opportunity to heal itself. In Quantum Neurology® Rehabilitation, I've mapped out the Nervous System through its experience ranges. I use traditional methods of neurological analysis combined with unique evaluations that I have developed. This allows me and my students to evaluate the Nervous System with the gold standard of neurological evaluations that is taught to every doctor around the world. Additionally, my patented system of neurological analysis allows us to find and correct hidden weaknesses within the Nervous System that are not found by other methods.

We now know many of the Nervous System indicators responsible for health and quality of life. It is our experience that, when these indicators are strengthened, the Nervous System expands. In its expansion, we see its restoration and healing. We can consistently restore function, strength and coordination. The same rehabilitation concepts that help athletes break world records are used to recover patients from paralysis. I have also developed techniques to restore lost sensation. We have had considerable success in restoring areas of numbness throughout the body, even in cases where the person had been damaged decades prior.

The principles applied to recover movement and sensory loss can be adapted to rehabilitate specific conditions. We strengthen areas of the Nervous System that are collapsed by injury, illness, infection or condition. We have consistently found once these areas are strengthened the body heals itself. It has been our experience that most people respond favorably to rehabilitation as long as the Nervous System is intact and demonstrates the ability to recover. This is usually evident within the first few sessions.

We have patients that have gotten up out of their wheel chairs, recovered from chronic illnesses, and recovered from strokes, brain injuries and paralysis. People have restored their vision from blindness, others have let go of their hearing aids. We have seen people achieve the highest levels of human performance, world records and gold medals. Others who were living in pain for years have become pain-free in a very short period of time. All of this has occurred by cultivating and expanding the Nervous System.

Our Nervous System is the completeness of who we are as humans—our entire body and being. When we evaluate the Nervous System, we look at its various layers of expansion or collapse.

An example of a collapse would be if we gave a peanut to somebody who had a severe allergy (anaphylaxis) to peanuts. You can visualize that person disconnecting from the universe as you witness the collapse of the Nervous System. The airway would shut down; the face would disconnect and go numb. The body loses its pressure sense as it starts to swell. The connection to the universe is lost through the sensation of the face and limbs. The absence of oxygen, which is necessary for universal connection, causes the person to turn blue. These are the signs of losing one's connection to the space around the body, the universe. Full disconnection is physical death.

The cultivation and expansion of the Nervous System is the opposite of the severe allergic reaction. Continuing where I left off in the example above, cultivating the Nervous System from damage is demonstrated through its ability to connect and integrate with our surrounding universe. Restoring the Nervous System would reverse the damaging effects caused by the anaphylaxis. Using this example as a model for the healing process, we consider the body's ability to reconnect the sensation of the face and open the airway to receive oxygen. The body would continue healing itself and recover from any damage caused by the lack of oxygen. Once the Nervous System was healed to its previously "normal" capacity, expansion would include the ability to introduce peanuts into this person's life without the Nervous System collapsing. Ultimately we would want to see the person's ability to thrive in the presence of peanuts (no longer an allergen). Once you can appreciate this concept, it is easier to recognize that your five senses are your direct connections to the universe and that its range of function relates to your quality of life.

We use the concept of expansion and collapse to restore the Nervous System from damage. I have developed methods to integrate physical movement of the body; I also integrate sensation, mental processing and organ function. Many of these concepts are advanced, or only have clinical applications, but the key is that they can be activated and stimulated to maximize the body's opportunity to heal.

Nervous System Layers

The Nervous System is best understood in layers. We have layers of function and different layers of communication. We have cellular, tissue, muscular, mental, person-to-person and spiritual communication. When there is Nervous System damage, we lack the ability to connect and communicate on one or more of these layers. In Quantum Neurology® we find the layer that is not communicating properly and stimulate the Nervous System to reintegrate itself and expand.

We rebuild the Nervous System in layers. Our goal is to strengthen the Nervous System to a level that stress and everyday wear and tear will never surpass. The amount of stress needed to cause injury is referred to as the *injury threshold.* Just as you would determine the maximum weight you can lift before hurting yourself during exercise, our goal is to increase the Nervous System's ability to handle stress. Stress can present through various physical, chemical and emotional burdens on the Nervous System. One would think that we expand the Nervous System by working the person to their highest threshold level of strength to expand their injury threshold. That is not the case; actually the integration is achieved layer by layer, function by function. Your abilities to handle intense pressure, cold, heat or various other Nervous System functions are integrated and contribute to you body's overall expansion. Some of the benefits of the Nervous System expansion are increased strength and injury threshold.

One of the easiest ways to understand the layers of the Nervous System is to map out sensation. Sensation is a combination of feelings experienced when we are touched. This is a combination of sensitivity to pain, temperature, light touch, deep touch, pressure and body position. The experience of your skin being touched is a combination of these known experiences, and each layer contributes to your reality experience.

In our model of neurological rehabilitation, we can regain each of these layers individually. We literally rebuild the Nervous System by strengthening each layer of function and communication. These concepts expand beyond the sensation of the body. We also see this occur with muscular function, range of motion, complex movement and mental processing.

V. Our Nervous System Generates Our Reality Experience

"When you are courting a nice girl an hour seems like a second.
When you sit on a red-hot cinder a second seems like an hour.
That's relativity."
—Albert Einstein, Theoretical Physicist

Our Nervous System generates our reality experience from moment to moment. What we *perceive* to be real is generated by our Nervous System. I want to emphasize that our perception is generated by the Nervous System. I did not say that our perception is *not* a real experience.

You are indeed seeing what you are seeing, feeling what you are feeling, experiencing what you are experiencing. The way you see, feel and experience is generated by your Nervous System. *Life* is a layered set of experience ranges occurring through our Nervous System. The simultaneous experiences of vision, hearing, smell, taste and sensation contribute to our physical reality experience.

Your Nervous System's experience is generated by its ability to be integrated to the universe. We may occupy the same physical space as one another, but we each have a unique vantage point of the universe. That vantage point is yours and yours alone. No one can share it with you. Remember that the observer must be included to create an accurate measurement, and you happen to be the only observer from your vantage point. That vantage point is called a reality tunnel or holographic projection. We each experience the universe generated from our respective Nervous System's vantage point. These vantage points are *parallel universes* existing simultaneously while occupying the same space. We are physically bound to each other through our shared experience ranges. These experience ranges connect us with one another. An example of people who do not share the same experience ranges as the population are those on the autism spectrum. Their experience ranges are different from most people. Certain sounds, textures and thoughts initiate a different reaction than they would in most other people. It is often said that people on the spectrum live in their own world. I personally would say they live in their own universe with their Nervous Systems tuned to different experience ranges than ours.

Your five senses provide your integration with the physical universe. These senses provide the foundation you perceive as your physical reality. The quality of integration and communication with your surroundings determines your quality of life, your health and your ability to manifest. These rules create your reality. Your Nervous System mediates every action, reaction and function in your body. Everything you can think of that your body does is mediated by your Nervous System. All injuries, illnesses, infections and conditions cause a disconnection from the universe. And the disconnection from the universe can leave the body vulnerable to injury, illness, infection and conditions. Understanding how you connect with your universe allows you to create your reality from moment to moment.

Just like rebuilding layers of communication, as we described previously, rebuilding the sense of touch is also best described in layers. The main layers that contribute to your physical sensations are: pain, temperature, vibration, light touch, deep touch, pressure and body position. Sensation can be lost in one or more of these layers leaving the others intact. Using the vibration layer as an example, a vibration injury could result from a baseball player that hits a ball and the bat vibrates into his hands causing pain in his hands. A construction worker using a jack hammer all day long could suffer from a vibration injury causing pain throughout the body. Another example is somebody who rides a motorcycle that vibrates at a certain high rate and then experiences an auto accident. The Nervous System records the vibration rate as part of the injury. So, whenever the injured person experiences the same vibration rate in the future, it sets off an alarm in the body and delivers a signal of pain, dysfunction and decreased range of motion. Unless this alarm signal is interrupted, people can experience chronic pain, dysfunction and decreased range of motion for many years, if not the rest of their lives. This is how Nervous System communication can get caught in a pain loop triggered by one of the senses injured in a previous trauma.

These examples demonstrate that the Nervous System communicates through its experience. When we look at these communications, we know each of our experiences is unique through our respective Nervous Systems. There is no way for me to know if the sensation of brushing a feather over my skin is exactly the same experience you have on your skin. We have no way to understand it on that level, but we can understand that we each have a similar experience.

Many people have altered experiences. For example, people with a condition called *Reflex Sympathetic Dystrophy*, or *RSD*. This may be labeled with different names, but ultimately it comes down to a hyper sensitivity of one or more *layers* of sensation. People suffering with this condition do not experience the same *light touch* of a feather that you and I may experience. That feather on their skin is an excruciating, unbearable, level ten out of ten lightning bolt type pain. They do not register the same experience that you and I have to the same stimulus. So, they have an altered experience. That same person can be grabbed tightly over the same area and experience no discomfort whatsoever. Grabbing tightly communicates through a different layer of communication called *deep touch*. The layer for *deep touch* registers completely differently than the layer of light touch. But *light touch* to that same person on the same area would cause excruciating pain.

Pain syndromes such as RSD, fibromyalgia and chronic fatigue can be devastating to a person and his or her quality of life. To rehabilitate these patients, we have to train their Nervous Systems to have an appropriate experience to the offensive stimulus. This is done clinically and has demonstrated a high-level of success in helping people recover from these types of neurological problems.

We have ways to retrain the Nervous System to reset its function to an appropriate response. Parts of the body, the Nervous System, may have a hyper reaction to an allergen, as we discussed with peanuts, or a hyper reaction to a relatively mild stimulus – the touch of a feather. These hyper reactions can all be readjusted through Nervous System rehabilitation concepts. We've recovered neurological deficits in patients who were initially damaged over 70 years prior. When we look at the Nervous System in this way, we register our experiences in layers and each layer can be enhanced, improved and individually recovered.

VI. Traditional Nervous System Training

Traditionally, the Nervous System is considered to be the brain, spinal cord and the nerves up to the point of connection with its target tissue, organ, muscle or bone. That is a great way to label the physical parts of the Nervous System. But this simply describes the Nervous

System's hard wiring without considering its function. It reminds me of the time that most people believed the universe to be centered by the sun with only nine planets in its orbit. A short period of time later, the concepts of galaxies, black holes and parallel universes were discovered. We have similarly discovered a new frontier in the Nervous System. We have just begun to see the possibilities of using the Nervous System to strategically guide its own exploration.

Traditional Nervous System training defines the body as a collection of systems: digestive, nervous, circulatory, lymphatic and musculoskeletal. Doctors are trained that we are a collection of these systems. Although this traditional system's training does not explain how life is generated or experienced, it provides an excellent understanding of where things are located physically and how they function and relate to one another. These systems work together as a unit. We separate them simply for learning purposes.

To get this perspective, you have to step back and look at the Nervous System on a much larger scale and on a much smaller scale. The rules have to apply both scales. When we look at these concepts, we look at how the body communicates, not only through every one of these systems, but as a whole.

On a large scale, a large portion of our Nervous System is dedicated to movement and sensation. All muscle-based movement is referred to as *motor function*, and our *sensory experience* comes through our five senses.

Within the sensory experience, a significant amount of communication happens with our skin, through the sense of touch. Our skin is an integral part of our Nervous System, and it contributes a majority of our reality experience. Just think about it: your skin is in direct contact and receives constant communication with its surroundings. The sense of touch records pain, temperature, vibration, light touch, deep touch, pressure and body position. All of that combined with the other four senses of seeing, hearing, smell and taste generates your reality experience.

To get a better understanding of skin, we need to look at how it develops. The elements which develop into the skin and Nervous System start to form shortly after conception. When the sperm and the egg unite they eventually form three layers of tissue. These are called germ layers. Each layer becomes responsible for developing major sections of your body. The skin and the Nervous System are from the same germ layer. So, in my experience, the skin "is" the Nervous System. In fact, I believe that each organ and cell of the body should be included as the Nervous System because they function together as a complete system not in individual parts.

An organ is more than we were taught in school. We should not be limited by the concept that an organ is a well-formed mass of tissue. I am suggesting we begin to recognize that organs are specialized Nervous System tissue. Organs accomplish specialized functions just as the retina is specialized tissue used in vision. This perspective allows us to reconsider the definition of an organ. Any time a group of cells, regardless of their location in the body, communicates in unison to perform a common action, it should be considered a holographic organ. Cells perform multiple duties and belong to multiple holographic organs. Holographic again refers to the body's nonphysical "software" communication. Blood is a liquid organ with examples of holographic communication through its oxygen levels, pressure, volume, infection and detox response. Other examples of holographic organs are bone marrow and adipose tissue. Each of these tissues is found throughout the body yet works in perfect unison regardless of its location.

While each cell, organ and tissue is connected to your body, in reality each is an independent living structure within you. Each works independently and yet, at the same time, each works together in unison to generate your life and your experiences. My life holds more meaning when I think of it this way. *Life* is a meaningful arrangement played through our Nervous System. Just like a symphony of well-trained musicians, each producing a unique sound in unison to create music, each cell projects its unique light in harmony and unison to project your *Life's* experience.

Chapter 4

KEY #2: WE ARE PROJECTIONS OF LIGHT

"Take it slowly. This book is dangerous!"
—From the book Fox in Socks by Dr. Seuss

Holograms are projections of light.

The second key to Nervous System Consciousness is having an understanding that we, too, are projections of light.

The light which we project has multiple layers of intelligence. Physically, we project our body image. Nonphysically, we project our mind, spirit, intentions and love. These Nervous System concepts can be explained within a holographic model.

The ability to communicate nonphysically through light makes us holographic beings. This means that our existence, *Life* as we know it, is a projection of light through our Nervous System. The hallmarks of holographic communication exist in us, in nature and in all living things. Observing this communication gives us insight into how we can access our Nervous System's holographic healing.

Now, let's see the holographic model of healing and how consciousness exists within the LightBody.

I. If We Are Projections of Light, Where Is the Projector?

Our experiences record the sensations we perceive from our internal, external and nonphysical environments. These experiences include all communications within our bodies, and nonphysically in our thoughts, emotions and our spiritual connections.

We are holographic beings because our Nervous System generates our *Life* experience through light. We are holographic light projections. Each and every cell of the body projects light. A key hallmark of a hologram is that all the information to create the hologram is contained within its smallest unit.

To understand how each cell's light projection contributes to our hologram, let's focus on the body and how it's constructed. The building block of the body is the cell. Of the trillions and trillions of cells in the body, every cell has the genetic material we refer to as DNA. The DNA can be removed from one cell, placed into another cell, pulsed with electricity and a copy of the original cell can be generated and developed into a full body in a procedure called cloning. This procedure is hot in ethical debates. Without getting into the ethics of this issue, cloning demonstrates that we are holographic beings. The cell, our smallest unit, contains all the information necessary to create an entirely new body.

Most cells in our body are round, so if you take a lot of round things and you pile them up, what shape do you get? You should get a mound shape. So, how are our bodies shaped the way they are? Given that we're made from trillions of little round things, why aren't we mound-shaped or at least round? I'm suggesting that these little round things collect and connect together, and they communicate to each other with light that projects from their DNA.

Fritz-Albert Popp, PhD discovered that each cell emits light from its DNA called a biophoton. The biophoton exhibits intelligent communication that travels at the speed of light from cell to cell and from cell to entire body.

The biophoton that is emitted is used for intelligent communication. I believe that this communication controls and mediates the nonphysical information of the body. Communication happens instantly through the cloud of intelligent light generated by each cell. Every cell shares its intelligent cloud of light with neighboring cells, each contributing its own projected light. Scientifically, this is referred to as the biophotonic field (bio – life, photon – light). I call the collective cloud of intelligent light communication generated from the trillions and trillions of cells of our body the *LightBody*. The LightBody coordinates all the cells of the body. It is through this nonphysical light network that our Nervous System can manage the complexity of communication necessary to exist with consciousness, kindness and intelligence.

I believe the LightBody is who we truly are. It is our essence, our spirit, our soul, our light. It houses nonphysical thoughts, concepts of self, spiritual connections and the ability to connect with the universe. The LightBody carries all these nonphysical attributes and abilities that we associate with our body or identity. All of this communication occurs through the light generated from the sum total of the entire body's trillions of cells.

If I asked you who you are, how would you describe yourself? Most people would list nonphysical attributes and say something like, "I'm a good person. I am loyal. I love my family. I trust my spiritual connection. I enjoy teaching and sharing with others." These are examples of nonphysical attributes.

Expanding this concept we must include what Dr. Sigmund Freud referred to as your *Id,* or your sense of self, as well as your mind, thoughts, capacity for joy, love and emotion. The LightBody is the hologram your cell's DNA projects which then generates the nonphysical you. All of your nonphysical attributes are suspended in this biophotonic field of light generated by the trillions of cells that make up your body which I am calling the LightBody.

II. Our LightBody

Our physical body is simply a lantern for the LightBody to exist. Your intellect observing these words exists because of your physical body's ability to interact with your nonphysical self. There must be a bridge that connects the physical and the nonphysical. In the Christian tradition, Jesus teaches that the body is the Temple. I believe that our physical body is a lantern or temple that generates and houses the nonphysical LightBody. The LightBody carries all the nonphysical Nervous System information suspended in its hologram.

Consciousness exists in your LightBody. Did you know that there is no direct connection between a part of your brain and your specific memories? There is no location in your brain, or your Nervous System, that is responsible for childhood memories. Science has not found a part of your brain that is responsible for riding a bicycle. They cannot pinpoint what part of your brain is responsible for the capacity for love, thought, emotion, or any one feeling.

For example, people may think that if the area above the ears—called the temporal lobe—is responsible for speech, that's where speech is located. In my experience, this is where the *information is processed* from the nonphysical holographic field into the physical Nervous System. Damaging a physical area of the body limits its ability to connect with the holographic field for speech communication. Damaging the physical connection of speech within the Nervous System does not remove the information from the field of the LightBody; the damage only limited the LightBody's ability to physically express the information.

We see people who have suffered traumatic brain accidents and partial losses of their brains are able to communicate fully and experience everything they experienced before, with less brain matter. We have also seen people remember their lives in its complexity after significant head injuries. Head injuries or dementia that result in amnesia can remove time frames, personalities, characteristics or individuals from a person's memory. A chunk of someone's brain could be missing and yet their childhood memories may be intact.

Your memories and knowledge are not as well defined as an individual brick. If a piece of the brain were removed, it would not remove well-defined pieces of knowledge. We can remove the pages of words beginning with the letters *Q*, *R* and *S* from a dictionary, yet a person with a head injury will not lose the memory of things starting with those three letters.

These situations demonstrate that the mind does not access information in a linear fashion. Just as moving an antenna will enhance or prevent you from accessing a radio or television signal, inability to access the hologram is a sign of Nervous System disconnection. We lose the ability to access our holographic information as the body physically deteriorates and loses its ability to connect to the holographic field.

The LightBody concept is not new although my description of it may be unique. We talk about it in our everyday life when we describe situations and people with these attributes. We talk about how certain people shed light on a subject, or they bring light to your life. An intelligent person is referred to as bright or brilliant. When a woman is pregnant she is said to be glowing or radiant. When someone dies the light leaves the body. These are common examples of the LightBody. Our body's light is emitting at a level we can perceive. This is not limited to the visual spectrum, but rather it occurs in a spectrum that is visible to our Nervous System.

In many traditions, light is synonymous with God. Light is synonymous with loving, healing, kindness and enlightenment. Light is the key to consciousness and is how we share this meaningful experience with each other. Just as each cell projects light that extends beyond its physical boundaries, the LightBody is formed deep within the body and extends past the physical frame. I believe the light that extends past the physical body reaches outward and literally plugs the body into the universe, the space around the body. It is the body's ability to generate a quality of light and brilliance that connects us to the Universe.

If you damaged part of your physical body (a broken hand), your body lantern would not be able to generate maximum LightBody for that area. You would experience limited healing and limited ability to connect the layers of communication in that area of your body (for example: sensation, strength and dexterity). You would experience pain, decreased sensation and a lack of function and physical control. You couldn't get that part of your body to perform actions with your mind because the connection would be damaged.

In Quantum Neurology®, we use Nervous System expansion principles to stimulate the body's natural ability to generate light in the damaged areas and to stimulate its healing using light therapy. The secrets to our amazing rehabilitation success have been in rehabilitating and strengthening the Nervous System with light. This has become our central focus.

In studying teachings of enlightened people, most share the concept that everyone and everything is connected in one consciousness. This concept fits into the Holographic Nervous System model, too. Again, I emphasize that light is consciousness. The light that extrudes through our Nervous System exhibits our innate and mental intelligence. We share our experience through light. We see each other through the visual spectrum of light. It is possible to master your ability to communicate more profoundly through the different layers of connection in the universe.

The nonphysical Nervous System is not limited by space, distance or time. When we look at memory and its accessibility, we can recall an endearing childhood experience that may bring tears to our eyes like it happened in the moment. That moment, even though it may have happened 20, 30, 40, 50 or 60 years ago, strikes us in part of our Nervous System which happens in the moment. Therefore, there is no difference to the Nervous System between a moment that occurs "now" and a memory we re-experience.

When you lose a sense, all your other senses become heightened. Blind people develop keen hearing. Some blind people even develop a sonar ability. They can walk around a room by listening to the sounds bouncing off the physical objects surrounding them. A blind person can also develop a keen sense of touch. Just looking at Braille can be intimidating and is a reality most people choose to ignore. I recommend you touch it each time you see it. Remind yourself that there is a way of communication through the sense of touch. Hopefully, you'll never have to learn Braille, but it's important to know that it's there.

Projected Shape

When one part of us is removed, whether through amputation or injury, we still have our complete memories of that life. What many don't realize is that, because we are holographic, the piece of the body that was removed has all the memories, too.

If we look at a Kirlian photograph of a leaf, we can see the outline of the leaf's bioenergetic field. When a corner of the leaf is cut off and then re-photographed, the original outline of the leaf's entire bioenergetic field is still visible, as if the leaf were completely intact. This is also observed in Kirlian photographs of lizards that have had their tails amputated. This holographic projection of light is created by cells of the entire human body as well. Humans with amputated limbs have taught us that they can maintain a sense of position, movement and sensation in the amputated limb or limbs. They often experience *phantom pain,* which are sensations registered by the Nervous System, as coming from the area of the removed limb or limbs. In this example, the remaining cells of the body generate a holographic projection of the entire human frame.

Normally the cells contributing to this holographic field assume the entire shape of the holographic projection, just as the amputated leaf or lizard's tail. Our trillions and trillions of cells assume the shape of their own holographic projection. This is why our cells do not pile into a mound shape or a shapeless blob on the floor. Our cells, from conception until death, generate the nonphysical holographic projection of our selves. These same cells then occupy the space created by that projection. It is the Nervous System's ability to generate and maintain this holographic projection that allows us to grow, heal and maintain our connection to the universe.

No Time or Space

The LightBody is the nonphysical part of our Nervous System. The nonphysical is not limited in the way that physical objects are limited. When we say something is physical it has three dimensions: length, width and height. It's easy to understand something physical as anything that can be measured with a ruler. Einstein taught us that *time* cannot be separated from the three dimensions of space. Physical space occupies time. In other words, if something is physical, and can be measured, it occurs in a moment of measurable time. The interaction of light expressed through our physical Nervous System, generates and records our *Life* experience through the collection of moments that generate the passage of time.

We can visualize this by using a clay extruder analogy. A clay extruder is a common toy that presses a ball of clay though a "die mold" shaped disc. The shape on the disc defines the clay expression. So, a circle shape on the die mold will make a long string of clay spaghetti. A rectangle will make a flat clay noodle. A human-shaped die mold will make a long, human-shaped clay string. The formed clay represents light and the passage of time as observed through the vantage point of the human-shaped die mold. The moment of "now" occurs as light (clay) passes through the DNA represented by the human-shaped die mold. *Life* is light extruded through your Nervous System and can be referred to as a reality tunnel or *holographic projection*. The reality tunnel is visualized by the string of human-shaped clay (light) formed by the human-shaped die mold.

Die Mold and Nervous System: The Moment of Now

If we take this a step further, let's line up an infinite series of clay extruders. Each clay extruder uses the die mold shape of a human. Each die mold represents an individual human Nervous System. The string of human-shaped clay (formed from each extruder) symbolizes the passage of light over time from each human's (die mold) perspective. When we observe the series of extruders, we see the individuality of each Nervous System and the clay string (reality tunnel) generated.

What makes this difficult to understand is that people are not toy extruders that shoot out clay (light) in one direction. Our Nervous System generates light that expands in *all directions*. A more accurate visualization of reality would be to line up an infinite series of light bulbs. Each light bulb represents a person from which light is emitted in all directions. Each light bulb becomes an observer in its own reality tunnel (holographic projection). We each have a shared reality experience because the light from each bulb occupies the same space. Our individuality is best observed in the clay extruder analogy, while our Holographic Nervous System is best observed in the light bulb analogy. The multiple individual Holographic Nervous Systems can be described as *parallel universes* occurring simultaneously and occupying the same space.

Hopefully this makes sense to you and you're starting to recognize that you are living a quantum (light) experience. The Nervous System is truly amazing. As we understand the Nervous System, we maximize human potential. We each have our own magnificent gem. Everyone simply needs to be taught what the Nervous System is and how to care for it properly. When people recognize that their central focus should be Nervous System cultivation and expansion, we will see humanity shift and watch the healing of populations overnight.

A new concept is displayed in how your physical body intertwines with the energetic body. This describes how your physical body generates its energetic body, and how the energetic body connects with your surrounding universe. The LightBody is your communication channel between the physical and nonphysical. Communication happens through the LightBody which is the culmination of light generated by every cell of the body.

The LightBody projects outward just as a light bulb's energy expands outward. If we dim the LightBody, and it retracts within the physical boundaries of the skin, we will see a shift in muscular strength and sensory perception. Within the field of neurology, we call this shift an *inhibition*. An example is the way that athletes and coaches describe muscles. They often say the muscle is "firing" or it is "not firing." It is not that the nerve is cut and does not supply energy; it is simply active or it is not active. That is an easier way to understand the word inhibition. When we say that a certain muscle is not firing, it is not getting its energy, it is not fully active. Using the concepts of the Holographic Nervous System, the body is literally unable to generate maximum LightBody or light in that area, so it is inhibited (not firing). The example of muscles firing or not firing explains the concept of inhibition. To describe the rest of the Nervous System, however, I prefer the concept of the *dimmer switch* (rheostat) for a light fixture. This concept is easy to visualize and applies to the entire Nervous System. Visualizing a full connection between a nerve and an organ as vibrant and thriving tissue, and zero connection between a nerve and an organ is gangrenous, dead tissue. It is not simply an on-off switch as described in the muscle example because a range of damage occurs between healthy tissue and death. *Firing* and *not firing* simply does not capture the fullness of that range. The *dimmer switch* concept allows people to understand that there is a range of connectivity directly proportional to health.

When the LightBody is dimmed, that area of the body has difficulty receiving sensory information. It can't perceive the pain, light touch, pressure and other information. The LightBody is responsible for carrying that information throughout the Nervous System. When that circuit is dim, just like a dim light in your dining room, it does not mean the light is off, it is simply too dim. When damaged, the Nervous System receives a dimmed signal of sensation compared to a full signal.

Nervous System Integration

In Quantum Neurology®, we simply reintegrate the Nervous System's ability to generate its light. We use the Nervous System's own intelligent guidance. The way the Nervous System guides us is simple. If we are working with a muscle that is not firing, we look for a way to stimulate the body that makes that muscle fire. This concept is simple when properly applied to the Nervous System and delivers tremendous healing.

The bottom line is...

*When you strengthen the Nervous System,
the body will heal itself!*

This is a premise of all natural healing. Chiropractic philosophy is based on Nervous System stress relief. I want to bring the public's understanding of the Nervous System into the new century. I have explored its boundaries and found unlimited healing resources within the Nervous System.

In the movie *Star Trek* there are different depictions of healing in the future. We are not far from that kind of activity. Today, I teach doctors how to use tools that are hovered over the body, stimulating the Nervous System. Light therapy demonstrates the ability to activate immediate neurological changes without even touching the body. But the important thing to remember is that machines and technology do not heal—it is your Nervous System that heals. The power that made the body heals the body!

We demonstrate this experience with certainty and teach it to other people so they can duplicate and validate it for themselves. It is exciting. When you look at the body this way, you start recognizing that this concept of neurological rehabilitation reintegrates the holographic communication of the body. As doctors, this changes our perception of who we are and what we are capable of doing to help rehabilitate the Nervous System.

I ask you to share these concepts with your friends and loved ones. Simply by understanding the concept of the LightBody, you can make educated life decisions. Using your intuitive guidance you can center yourself with every thought, food consumed or action taken. You decide what contributes to your Nervous System's ability to generate its LightBody. My goal is to teach every single person and every doctor the concepts of Nervous System cultivation and expansion.

Our bodies have done this all along. What is new is our ability to focus on the interconnection between the physical body and the energetic body. We may never understand it entirely, but within these new concepts, we can understand ourselves more profoundly.

Chapter 5

KEY #3: HEALING THE HOLOGRAPHIC NERVOUS SYSTEM

"Medical Miracle: The unexplained spontaneous regression of a medical condition thought to be invariably fatal or incurable or both."
—Taber's Cyclopedic Medical Dictionary, 16th edition

If we were to study all the miracle healing events ever documented, the miraculous healing has been attributed to various reasons. In Christian and other religious traditions, healing is an act of God. In modern science, it is called *spontaneous regression* or *spontaneous healing*. Regardless of where you are in your beliefs of miraculous healing, I want everyone to agree on one thing—the Nervous System was healed. It does not matter to what we attribute the healing. We each possess the most powerful healing instrument in the universe. It is important to recognize that miraculous healing is available through the Nervous System.

I. The Arrogance of Science

There are good and bad elements in all professions. What I call the *arrogance of science* demonstrates the thought forms that permeate the chemical health industries. The population is so ingrained in the profit-based education provided by the chemical health industries that they have difficulty looking into new concepts that do not originate within the chemical care model. Many modern scientists and governments around the world, as well as the patients who are treated, have blindly adopted a locked-in position regarding science.

We Know Everything There Is to Know

The chemical industry, in its arrogance, has a blind spot that exists in two forms. The first is: "We know everything there is to know." The second: "Everything that is known has always been known." This arrogance happens in every era. When bloodletting and other barbaric therapies were the best science available at that time, these techniques were widely practiced. Those doctors were not bleeding their patients with the intent to harm; they actually thought they were doing good. Although it's hard for us to imagine, there must have been people that demanded bloodletting to be performed on themselves and loved ones even after it was commonly understood that it didn't help heal the body.

We have advanced past bloodletting practices, but barbaric medical techniques are still commonplace around the world. The modern day "health care" industry is a business that often limits its services to profitable methods of cutting, burning or poisoning the population instead of profitable and cost effective ways to heal the population. We see the "health care" industry, with all its investors, beneficiaries and employees, profiting by perpetuating the patients' dependencies on products and services. As technology escalates, it will soon be impossible to afford care in this model.

Over 60 percent of bankruptcies in the United States list high medical expenses as contributing to their financial difficulties. In 2000, the World Health Organization ranked the U.S.A. health care system first in responsiveness, highest in cost, 37th in overall performance and 72nd in overall level of health. To state it simply, the U.S. population is being overcharged for unnecessary medical and chemical services. People will have no choice but to care for themselves and seek doctors outside of the industrialized chemical and medical systems. Individuals must find experts to care for their families in supporting, strengthening and expanding their Nervous Systems.

We do not live in a sterile environment, and we are not supported or healed by the volumes of toxic chemicals that are dumped into our bodies, air, food, water or our environment. We are all aware of insurance companies declining patients' care for profit reasons. Anonymous decision makers within insurance offices, who have never seen or examined patients, are responsible for dictating the patients' available care. Just talking about this method of care is horrific. The current model is very different from the holographic Nervous System model I described in the last few chapters. Unfortunately, the world will be locked into the current model of "health care" until its financial collapse, or the population reaches its tipping point and demands a new model.

The current model of health care is failing. We are coming to a point in society where the mind-set is going to make a huge shift. The people who do not get this information will be vulnerable to being subjected to the health care created to support the shareholders' bottom line.

We need to shift the population's focus from the chemical management of life, to a life free of chemicals. Imagine if we could elevate the population to become Nervous System conscious. Imagine a population that uses the Nervous System to guide its care. Imagine it being basic knowledge that when things collapse your Nervous System they are bad for you, and when things expand your Nervous System they are good for you. Imagine a population that recognizes how thoughts, foods, actions and people directly affect the Nervous System, and uses this knowledge as a guide to a happier, healthy and conscious *Life*. Imagine a population that focuses on Nervous System cultivation and expansion. Imagine the businesses and products that would flourish in this mind-set. I look forward to the world's consciousness being elevated through this model of thought and understanding.

With today's technology, it is easier to generate a new reality than ever before. We can master absolutely anything we want to learn. The number of people going from pauper to billionaire within one lifetime is increasing. Your ability to direct your reality is far more powerful than you may have been taught. Once you learn to focus the reality your Nervous System generates, you can then direct and steer your reality experience —your *Life*.

Everything That Is Known Has Always Been Known

In 1628, William Harvey, an English physician to Charles I, presented his research on the motion of the heart and blood. He was the first to introduce the concept of the circulatory system as we know it today. We take this basic health knowledge for granted. Imagine living life without that information. How different would reality be? We all grew up knowing that the heart pumps blood through arteries and veins, yet prior to his discovery, science thought the heart was a heater, and that the arteries and veins were there to cool off the heat generated by the heart. This is probably why bloodletting was a common practice. If the heart were a heater and a person had a fever, draining the hot blood to cool off the body may sound like a good idea. It only sounds like a good idea if you believe the heart is a heater. Through painstaking research and dissection, Harvey mapped out and accurately described the circulatory system as we know it today. He emphasized that the key to his research and discovery was studying the heart in living subjects as opposed to dead subjects. It took nearly 50 years of public ridicule by his peers before his work was recognized.

The second component to the arrogance of science is: "everything that is known has always been known." The day before William Harvey presented his work, people did not have a clear understanding of the circulatory system. Even after he presented it, the doctors and the public did not completely understand his model. If we imagine that each person is a cell projecting his or her mind-set about the circulatory system into society, the society's knowledge was locked on the heart-heater concept. It took 50 years for that mind-set to shift. Then, it became common knowledge, "Of course there is a circulatory system that is pumped by the heart. You didn't *know that?*" we now gasp.

The arrogance of science is the attitude that everything there is to know is already known. If you speak to an educated, science-minded person, at times you may get the response, "If I'm not familiar with the concept, or if I haven't heard of it—it does not exist," or "If I did not invent it myself, it is not real or valid," or "If it does not have a double-blind placebo-controlled study that has been peer-reviewed and published in a premier medical journal (sponsored by the chemical industry)…it's not worth my time." In the intellectual game of "I'm a doctor, so I know it all," it is easy to get stuck in thinking that because you are really good at what you do, and you know so much about your area of expertise, that there is nothing left for you to learn. This attitude is often encountered in really high-level scientific-minded people. Professionally, you may feel much more vulnerable to acknowledge what you do not know or understand clearly, but being vulnerable and always wanting to learn more is truly a strength.

There is danger in this superior mind-set and its ability to abuse patients and the public. This mind-set makes people feel inferior if they question or disagree with what is being presented, especially if the concept is supported by an expert in a field they know little about. If you didn't know…you're an idiot! If you disagree…you're an idiot! If you don't buy their chemicals, you're an idiot! If you don't do as you're told … you're an idiot!

YOU are NOT an idiot! You have been manipulated, domesticated and brainwashed by professional marketing campaigns that benefit chemical industries by profiting and gaining power from your illnesses.

Modern industries have brainwashed the population into ignorance. We have been domesticated and educated through media advertising and marketing funded primarily by chemical and medical industries. For many consumers, most, if not all, of their health knowledge comes directly from commercials, sitcoms and "reality" television.

We have been trained to seek convenience at the expense of our health, time and quality of life. The chemical and medical industries are well aware of how the body and mind work. They know how to press your buttons and make you consume what you don't need.

It's time to take action. Wake up from the delusion generated by the television and media that is primarily funded by the chemical and medical industries. The easiest way to stop participating in the delusion is to *stop watching television programming*. It's called programming for reason.

Being aware is the first step to gain full control of your mind and body! Once you remove the constant bombardment of television and media from your thoughts, you may have an amazing experience: your own thoughts and beliefs, which are not based on what the talking heads on television told you to think, will begin to surface.

Removing television and media from your thoughts will free your mind to heal your body. With this new available head space, you can focus on the issues and emotions that have held you back from living the most amazing life possible, starting with the most volatile illusion...pain!

II. The Three Illusions: Pain, Dysfunction and Decreased Range of Motion

If our Nervous System is so wonderful, why does it generate pain? I agree that a life without excruciating or chronic pain would be a good way to go, but our Nervous System needs a way to protect and warn us against harmful things that disconnect the Nervous System from the physical universe.

Our Nervous System has three ways to protect us from damaging ourselves. I call them *The Three Illusions*: pain, dysfunction and decreased range of motion. These are nonphysical restraints that our Nervous System uses to protect us by automatically alerting, activating or deactivating certain functions. If we reset the Nervous System's hologram, the illusion can disappear...immediately!

Pain Does Not Exist—Pain is an Illusion!

I've had heated discussions over this statement many times. It's not the easiest thing for a person who may be in chronic excruciating pain to hear.

Pain is not physical. Pain is an illusion because it cannot be removed from your body—we cannot remove the pain signal from our body, put it in a box and send it to somebody we don't like. Pain is not a synthetic chemical deficiency. It's a holographic illusion generated by the Nervous System.

I'm not denying that you or anyone experiences pain. It's important to know that pain is not the problem; it's only a signal, a messenger. Before telephones, during war, communication between enemies was handled via personal messenger. This is where the phrase "don't kill the messenger" comes from.

Pain is your Nervous System's messenger. Pain is not your enemy; pain is your guide. We use the pain signal as one of many methods of validating the patient's healing experience. When a person's condition is improving, their pain symptom is often relieved. Pain is a symptom not a cause. Chemicals do not take away pain; they only block your body's ability to recognize what is wrong. In many cases, when the Nervous System recognized that its message is being blocked, it will strengthen the message and create more pain to override the chemicals blocking the message (signal). I am not against using pain blocking medications; I am simply saying that chemicals used to block pain do not correct the problem that created the pain signal.

We see evidence in a common example that the pain signal is not the source of the problem. Have you ever tried shutting off another person's obnoxiously loud cell phone? If you can reach it, but you're not familiar with the model, press any button, bang on it and throw it on the floor—it doesn't shut off. More likely the sound is nearby, and you can't get your hands on the phone. You could try swinging your hands through the air, to no avail, or cover your ears to stop the sound. The sound may hurt your ears, but it's only the signal. It's the messenger not the enemy. The signal, the sound that delivers the pain, is not the cause of the problem. The problem is the phone, and it will drive you crazy if you can't shut it off.

Many of today's medical solutions offer the same misguided model: fix your ears instead of correcting the source by shutting off the phone. Treat the symptom, not the cause. Just as the sound of a cell phone ringing is not located where you feel it on your body (your ears), your Nervous System can deliver pain signals to any area within the body. This is called *pain referral*. It's easy to recognize local pain. If you were to break your finger, you would know exactly where it hurts with pinpoint precision. It is not so obvious when pain is generated from non-traumatic or organ problems.

A common example of *pain referral* is seen during a heart attack. It is said that the first sign of a heart problem is often death, because people have not been trained to recognize the pain referral of the heart and don't take corrective action before heart attack begins.

Internal organs and glands such as the heart do not have sensation ability. If I were magically able to reach into your chest and pinch your heart, it would not feel the same as a pinch on your skin. Your heart and other organs lack the sensitivity and pain reception of the skin. When an organ is under stress it will pull energy from the resources that share the same nerve supply. The shared muscle, tissue, organs and bones will be stressed from the energy pull of the distressed organ (heart). When an organ or gland is under stress, the Nervous System delivers an alarm signal. All the functions sharing that the same nerve (wire) will signal distress (pain, numbness, cramping or dysfunction). Each nerve wire, when under stress, will deliver a *pattern of dysfunction,* also known as *pain referral.* In the heart example, the main pain referral pattern follows the nerve wires called C8 and T1 (C8 – 8th Cervical nerve, T1 – 1st Thoracic nerve). The pain referral symptoms along this nerve wire include tightness, numbness and pain in the areas of the chest, left arm, shoulder, neck and jaw with a clenched fist, heavy sweating and difficulty breathing. There may be nothing wrong with areas along the heart's nerve wire. The neck, shoulder, arm and hand can be perfect, but when the distress signal is turned on by the heart, the victim will experience pain and numbness (pain referral) in those areas because they share the same nerve wire.

Nervous System Illusion #1: *Pain*

The first illusion, *pain,* is a signal created when your body is being disconnected from the universe, the space around your body. We each have a unique pain experience with consideration that my ability to tolerate pain is different from yours. The sensation is often rated from zero to ten, where zero is "no pain" and ten is a call for emergency help. Pain is necessary for survival. Without it we can die from inability to react or move away from a harmful stimulus such as fire or a sharp object. Regardless of how your pain compares with the pain others feel, when you look at your daily life and all the challenges that you face, I am sure you would agree that life is better when pain-free.

Pain is an illusion that your Nervous System generates to protect you. If you were to sprain your left ankle, it would be difficult to put your full body weight on the left foot because of pain. This pain is created by your Nervous System and protects you from taking further actions that can progress the injury. In the case of a physical injury, it is quite obvious you shouldn't step on the sprained ankle. It is more challenging when pain is not so obvious. When it can be initiated by so many non-traumatic or long-standing problems, it may be difficult to recognize the cause.

Using Quantum Neurology® Nervous System rehabilitation, my students and I see people many times a day in significant pain become pain-free. Clinically, we have used my techniques with light therapy to decrease and eliminate pain in a relatively short period of time. In some cases as quickly as five seconds. I do not take the pain away from the body. I simply stimulate the Nervous System in a particular fashion, that allows itself to communicate more efficiently and reset its pain signal. Having a deeper understanding of the Nervous System allows us to maneuver its reality (pain) experience.

Nervous System Illusion #2: *Decreased Range of Motion*

Continuing with the sprained ankle example we can look at the second illusion of decreased *range of motion*. Pain alone will limit your movement. Inflammation of the tissue creates a pressure splint around the ankle, limiting its physical ability to move through range of motion. Although in this example it is obvious that inflammation causes a physical barrier that blocks joint movement, inflammation is not necessary for the Nervous System to limit a joint's range of motion. The Nervous System has the ability to limit a joint's range of motion to an exacting degree. When the unnecessary protective mechanism is corrected the range of motion is often partially or fully restored— immediately.

Nervous System Illusion #3: *Dysfunction*

Having a limp from a sprained ankle can lead to back pain and other joint pains due to your body having to physically carry itself in an awkward manner to avoid the pain and compensate its movement in response to the decreased range of motion. The third illusion, Nervous System *dysfunction*, occurs in all areas associated to the injury. Each dysfunction is an added stress to the Nervous System which must be managed. The local tissue is affected by swelling and decreased circulation. The lymphatic system is stressed by moving more cellular debris out of the injured area. The bowel, bladder and sexual organs will share the burden of stress with the injured ankle because they share the same nerve wire. Incontinence, constipation and sexual dysfunction can all be associated to an ankle injury because of this shared nerve supply.

Understanding the three Nervous System illusions of *pain, decreased range of motion* and *dysfunction* is crucial for your health, development and self conservation. Your understanding of these mechanisms allows for the instant correction of many issues simply by resetting the Nervous System in the affected area. We are not curing the body of its affliction; we are activating the Nervous System to heal itself. When neurological connections are made we often see an immediate improvement in the patients' pain, range of motion and function.

Healing the body in this way may be new to you, but it is based in allowing your Nervous System to guide the healing. For some, this may be an obvious process of describing natural healing; others may benefit from a comparison between the biochemistry model of health with the holographic Nervous System model.

III. The Biochemistry Model

Most people are well aware of the biochemistry model of medicine, also known as Western medicine. This is the model most of us had our entire lives. The thought form of this model has been generated by industries that reap its benefits. This model is shared by most of the educated world. Outside of Eastern medicine, it is the primary method of analysis, evaluation and care for the world's population.

I will refer to the biochemistry model as a synthetic (or chemical) model. For the most part, the treatments are not based on natural healing processes. The use of synthetic chemicals is emphasized to *force* the body into an activity or action. Chemicals do not heal the body; they disconnect and destroy the Nervous System. Synthetic chemicals may numb the feeling your body experiences, or they may block the natural processes of your body. In other situations they stimulate an action.

At times, these synthetic chemicals may be necessary for emergency or temporary use. But I want you to clearly understand that synthetic chemicals do not belong in your body. You must reduce your body's synthetic burden. All synthetic chemicals must be processed through various parts of the Nervous System. If these chemicals can't be processed, they will be stored somewhere within the body. It takes valuable energy from your body to store and process these synthetic chemicals. When a person has more synthetic chemicals to store and process than energy available, he or she may experience chronic fatigue and chronic pain (fibromyalgia) type symptoms.

This biochemistry model makes our bodies into petri dishes. Our health is dictated from birth to grave by vaccines, chemicals and products that add unnecessary toxic chemical stress to the Nervous System. Synthetic chemical-based products, like antiperspirant, block your body's natural actions. It is natural for our bodies to sweat. If you block your body's natural ability to detoxify, over time, the congestion or stagnation of toxins can cause significant health problems. Imagine blocking your body's ability to urinate simply because you didn't like the smell of your urine.

Health problems are created when major channels of elimination are blocked. When caring for your body, be sure to completely avoid synthetic chemicals, especially on your skin, eyes, ears, nose, throat and private areas. As a general rule if you wouldn't put it in your mouth, it does not belong on your body. Avoid synthetic fragrances and cosmetics. Women are especially vulnerable to synthetic chemicals. Feminine hygiene products can contain synthetic chemicals and fragrances that irritate and contribute to chronic infection. You should only use organic, non-GM cotton, non-toxic and fragrance free products.

Adopt the attitude that anything that comes in contact with your body feeds your Nervous System. Remember, nutrients and vitamins come from food we eat and are also transferred from sunlight and absorbed by direct contact through our skin. Only allow your Nervous System to be in contact with things that nourish and expand it. This applies to all aspects of your Nervous System: physical, mental, emotional, financial, sexual, interpersonal and spiritual.

Keep Taking Your Meds!

I *do* want everyone to know that, in some cases, chemicals serve a purpose. In some cases, that purpose is life-sustaining or necessary to maintain quality of life. I want you to keep taking your prescribed medications ("meds") for as long they contribute to your quality of life. I cannot predict what meds you are taking and how quickly your body can heal. You may feel that you are helping your body by taking *synthetic* over-the-counter drugs, *synthetic* vitamins and *synthetic* prescription products, but these products only offer a *synthetic recovery*. A synthetic recovery alters the natural healing process by synthetic chemicals and artificial means.

Synthetic Chemicals Do Not Belong In Your Body!

Ultimately, when you use synthetic chemicals you damage your Nervous System's ability to heal itself naturally. Even when the product may be life supporting or provide symptomatic relief, consider how to manage the significant toxic burden that these chemicals place on your body. People are simply not aware of the dangers of synthetic chemicals. My recommendation is to completely remove synthetic chemicals from your life. This is challenging in today's society, but your goal should be to minimize your exposure to unwanted chemicals in your body.

Do Not Make Changes to Your Current Medications Without Consulting Your Doctor

There is no way to predict or guarantee how your body would respond to sudden shifts in your blood chemistry. You need to take responsibility for your Nervous System by informing yourself about your conditions and medications. If you are on medications and want to get off them, you will have to do your own research. Make a list of your medications, write what each is for, note the side effects, dosage, and note any food or drug interactions. Find out what your medications are made of and how they are made. Be aware that some medications can cause serious health and behavioral problems when stopped suddenly.

You deserve to know what you put in your body. With Internet access, answers are readily available. You may be surprised by the toxic burden that you're taking on simply to manage your symptoms. Work with your doctor, or find a doctor who will work with you, to decrease the synthetic chemical burden on your body.

Your goal should be to live a healthy life free of synthetic chemicals. I consider a healthy life one that is sustained by nature with the freedom to choose what goes onto or into my body. I, for one, am a firm believer in living, breathing and maintaining quality of life.

So, why is our health care based on managing prescriptions? Where are the programs that motivate people to be healthy and live a healthy, chemical-free life? Teaching a prescription-free lifestyle is not profitable for chemical industries. We deserve to be healthy and chemical-free. Our children deserve a life with unlimited access to healthy, organic foods, clean air and water. This delivers the building blocks of a healthy Nervous System.

When we look at the holographic Nervous System model of the body, we monitor its expansion and collapse to guide its healing. We use the expansion of the Nervous System to guide the care we provide during rehabilitation. We simply follow the Nervous System's recommendations of stimulation. We have seen consistently that, by doing this, the patient's body will heal itself.

IV. A Different Game Means Different Rules

Most people in the world have been raised in the Western medicine model of care. For many, it is the only care they know. It may be difficult for some to realize it is a model of thought with advantages, disadvantages, strengths and weaknesses; however, Western medicine is not the only model.

I want you to live a healthy amazing life. I want you to contribute your highest projection. To do that, and make educated choices, you need to know the rules of the game of life and death, health and illness.

I want to emphasize the differences between the chemical care model and Nervous System model. When using the Nervous System to guide care, we work with the Nervous System and amplify its natural healing. A sports analogy demonstrates why we see such amazing healing and recovery. The ultimate goal of helping a patient should be to get him or her to a healthy life—this is a win. The ultimate goal of playing a sport is also to win. Let's use the analogy of two different sports: hockey and baseball, where the exact way to win is different for each sport. In baseball, you have to run around the bases and come back to home base; in hockey, you have to score a goal. There are different tools, parameters and rules in each game. And, of course, hockey is played on ice versus running on grass, which changes the physics applied to the game. There are many differences between these two different models of play, yet each has the same goal—to win.

Which Game Do You Want To Play?

You are the observer in your universe. Your body is the object of interest (the ball) that keeps the game alive. It's your body—you get to choose the game: the chemical game, the Nervous System game, or both.

In Nervous System rehabilitation, the rules differ from those of the biochemistry model. First and foremost, you have to recognize that the Nervous System needs healing. This is not a priority in the biochemistry model. Instead, a Western evaluation is similar to how a mechanic would check a car needing maintenance or repair. Beginning with the fluids, a mechanic would check the oil, just as a doctor would do your blood work. Instead of checking the tires, the doctor will physically check the prostate (or vagina), squeeze the private parts and ask you to cough. It is an automotive type of physical approach to the body.

There is definitely the need for this type of physical evaluation, but you need to know that it is different from the performance-based evaluation used for neurological rehabilitation. The biochemistry model looks at synthetically shifting body chemistry to affect the body. In the Nervous System model, however, we check for how the body performs in its actions and reactions. We check every nerve function of the body in strength and sensation ability. We evaluate and strengthen how the Nervous System responds to a stimulus such as an allergen or fungus. Our corrections are done by stimulating the body to respond appropriately. Nothing is added and nothing is taken away.

I feel that you cannot heal the body by adding the burden of synthetic chemicals on top of what the body already has to process for the illness. The holographic Nervous System is very different. It is based on the rules of quantum physics. We use the holographic communication of the body to effect change within the Nervous System. The overall goal is to get the patient well. But, just as hockey and baseball have different physics that apply to how the games are played, different physics apply when we are healing the body. We activate the body's natural healing systems which demonstrate amazing regenerative abilities through this understanding.

V. The Holographic Transfer

Holographic transfer is a concept I developed for my father-in-law, Vicente Guzman. He was in the hospital with pancreatic cancer, and his cancer had spread to his liver and other organs. Pancreatic cancer is a silent killer. It does not demonstrate symptoms until it has spread throughout the body. Often, as in Vicente's case, there is not enough warning.

Prior to finding out about his cancer, Vicente had complained of low back pain. I worked on him to provide relief. He lived about an hour away, so he came in whenever he could. One day I worked on him and then we had lunch. Although his back felt better after our session, he was in pain again after lunch. He had managed diabetes for over 30 years, so it was not uncommon for him to reinjure himself. I worked on him again thinking that the food or his dessert at lunch may have stressed his

Nervous System and caused him to reinjure. After his second session, again, he had some relief, but within about 15 minutes, and without any additional stress, he experienced severe discomfort.

If It's Not Getting Better...It's Getting Worse!

In Nervous System rehabilitation we see so much success that it becomes a concern when people do not respond to care. I have a rule that I teach my doctors about a patient's rehabilitation: if it's not getting better, it's getting worse.

After a series of blood tests and imaging procedures, we discovered Vicente had developed pancreatic cancer that had already spread to various organs. With very short notice, his systems started to collapse. He was hospitalized with liver and kidney failure and going down quickly. The doctors at the hospital said there was nothing they could do. His liver looked like Swiss cheese and they were making him as comfortable as possible.

As a family, we strategically took shifts caring for Vicente in the hospital. We fed him fresh juices made from kale, spinach, celery and other dark green leafy vegetables to help alkalize his body and restore his pH. Vicente was a huge advocate of Quantum Neurology® and insisted I keep an out-of-state speaking engagement. I left knowing he was in good care with my family and I would return in a couple of days.

As my second father, Vicente has been one of the biggest supporters and contributors to Quantum Neurology®. He helped any way he could. He knew that his contribution, no matter how small or trivial, facilitated our helping countless others heal their bodies. He would come to the office, take out the trash, run errands and join us for lunch. He was so excited just to be there. He wanted to know about all the success stories in what was new and exciting in the frontiers of neurological rehabilitation.

I stayed in constant communication with Vicente and the family while I was out of town for the speaking engagement, but I sat in my hotel room frustrated that I could not help Vicente or be there to treat him. It was then the concept of the *holographic transfer* occurred to me. I posed a question to myself, "If illness is caused by an improper connection, or projection, of the LightBody, how can I remind his DNA what it should do to generate its *original projection?*"

The concept of reminding the DNA of its original projection would not leave my mind. If only I could remind his DNA of its original projection. The holographic transfer concept was born in this moment of necessity. I called Dan, Vicente's son, and asked him to use his own DNA sample (cells collected with a cotton swab rubbed on the inside of his cheek) to remind his dad's DNA of its original projection. I walked Dan through the procedure of holographic transfer over the phone.

The next morning I returned, and we performed *Holographic Transfer* again with the DNA cell samples collected from each of Vicente's children and grandchildren. It is a beautiful concept to know that a family can participate and heal each other using the hologram within their own DNA.

The holographic transfer concept reminds the body of its original projection. The DNA sample acts as a reminder to the Nervous System of its original glory. It is a good idea to keep samples of your entire family's DNA. This is how we remind the body of its original projection, to bring the memory of your Nervous System back to that of pre-injury or pre-illness condition. Ideally it is done with your own DNA, but if that is not available, you could use samples from one or both parents, siblings or your own children and grandchildren.

Once we activated the holographic transfer concept in his body, his DNA was reminded of its original projection. We did not know what to expect, so we continued to nourish his body with organic foods, whole food concentrates and raw vegetable juices. The juices supplied him with dense nutrients easily processed by the body.

The next day, Vicente's kidney levels went to normal function. His liver function improved by 50 percent. Vicente's health and energy improved so quickly he was discharged from the hospital the following day.

The holographic transfer allowed his body to pull from resources that were not available before. He had two good weeks after leaving the hospital where his Nervous System demonstrated amazing resilience. Most people with pancreatic cancer suffer incredible pain, but he could visit with family and say his final goodbyes. He passed away within six weeks of his diagnosis. I am so grateful that we could manage his pain with Quantum Neurology® and light therapy. He lived virtually pain-free until his transition. I wish I could tell Vicente that he was an inspiration for this valuable healing concept in Holographic Transfer.

Death is Inevitable—Health is Optional

Working with Vicente's circumstance was like trying to stop a loaded trailer truck from running off a cliff. We applied the brakes to slow the progression of his disease, but ultimately we ran out of road. Eventually everyone dies. I will die. You will die. Our families will die. Stop focusing on death. Instead, focus on creating and living the most amazing life possible.

Vicente was the biggest fan of Quantum Neurology® because it added value and quality to his life. It aided his recovery and management of various health issues, including diabetes. Nervous System rehabilitation accelerated his wound healing and restored multiple incidences of diabetic foot ulcers fully in a few weeks, his vision after multiple retinal detachment and inner eye bleeds, and lost sensation from peripheral neuropathy. I could go on, but the bottom line is that Nervous System rehabilitation amplifies the body's natural healing processes. It maximizes what is available within the Nervous System.

Holographic Transfer has quickly become one of the key principles of Quantum Neurology®. The ability to remind the Nervous System of its original projection has provided tremendous healing. Save samples of your entire family's DNA, preferably from the youngest or healthiest times of your life. *Any tissue sample can be used.* It does not take much to save a locket of hair (untreated, no chemicals), baby or adult teeth (without metals or amalgams on them). For now, save a current DNA sample until you find and store your earliest healthy DNA sample.

If you do not have access to your own DNA from a younger, healthier time in your life, you can use your healthy family's DNA. Current DNA samples can be used, but the youngest healthiest sample is best. Both parents' genetics contributed to creating your DNA, therefore one or both parents' DNA samples can be used. Siblings born of one or both parents will share genetics and can be used. The patients' children's DNA can also be used. Any tissue sample can be used but must be packaged and labeled for long term storage. Consider multiple storage locations such as a home fireproof safe, a safety deposit box, or both. Do this for your family and loved ones. Make a sample set for each family member to keep in a safe place wherever he or she lives. Ensure your family has access to its true wealth—the healthiest DNA sample. DNA holds the key to your family's future healing.

Chapter 6

KEY #4: HEALING WITH FOOD

"Let food be thy medicine, and let thy medicine be food."
—Hippocrates

The food chain does not include synthetic chemicals, hydrogenated fats, or anything produced or manufactured. Your holographic light projection is built from the light projection ability of the foods you eat. The Nervous System thrives when we nourish it properly and remove its toxic burden. When we strengthen the Nervous System, the body heals itself. To achieve the highest levels of living a healthy and energized life, and to manifest the highest projection of your LightBody, you must provide your Nervous System with the highest quality raw materials: *real food!*

I. Real vs. Synthetic

In our intelligence, we tend to forget we are animals. As most mammals, we share similar animal characteristics: live birth, born with hair (or fur), breathe oxygen and nurse our young. As all living organisms, we exist by eating other living things. For thousands of years, we humans thrived on eating plants and animals. This is how our body sustains itself.

We cannot sustain ourselves using synthetic, non-plant, non-animal based PHUDES. I purposely misspell the word *phude* to make the distinction that, while it may sound the same, it is synthetic. Phude is not real food! *Real food* refers to the edible and medicinal plants and animals that occur naturally on the planet. Pretty much anything living that grows from the ground or runs around can be eaten and is real food. The problem is that fewer people are eating real foods.

Once a food has been altered from its original raw state, it loses its nutrient value. Life-providing nutrients are destroyed once raw food is heated over 120° F. If nutrient destruction occurs simply by heating raw food, what nutrients do you think are available in highly processed and packaged phudes? Probably just the synthetic "fortified with" vitamins and minerals listed on the label.

Highly processed phudes are loaded with synthetic chemicals that do not occur naturally on this planet, making them synthetic phudes. These phudes are chemically engineered to fool our taste buds and pass as "food" but are far from real food that grows from the ground or runs around. Many chemicals used during the processing and manufacture of packaged phudes are known to cause serious illnesses. Beyond eating foods cooked from raw organic ingredients, avoid all phudes processed with chemicals.

To live a Nervous System conscious and healthy life a higher level of food discernment is necessary. Access to real food is the key to health. The most concerning example of synthetic phudes are indistinguishable from real food because they are "genetically modified" (GM). These synthetic phudes were engineered in a lab. The GM phudes contain DNA from various species of plants, animals, viruses or bacteria. They may look the same as your regular foods but they are synthetic. Synthetics are not natural to your body; they do not support or sustain life.

There is a difference between knowing *how to* support your Nervous System and *actually living* a lifestyle that supports your Nervous System. It can be challenging to take my recommendations to heart and live them day to day. We strive toward a goal of perfection, but even with all this information, we may fall short of perfect. The key is to forgive yourself. Acknowledge where you are in each moment, good or bad, and remind yourself of what you truly want for your life. With that positive attitude, remove the focus from your "failures," focus on what you want to accomplish and take action toward your goal.

You Can't Stop Eating

Food is a tricky subject. There is an overwhelming abundance of information and systems for eating. Even as a health professional, I managed to get really fat because I focused all my energy outside of myself. I gave all my time and energy to others and neglected myself. It was not until I focused on living according to simple principles that apply to any diet program that I regained my life and health. By simply shifting your habits ever so slightly, you can decrease your body's synthetic burden. One of the most important habits to develop is not *adding* chemicals to your foods.

Food Additives

The quickest way to decrease your synthetic burden is to avoid synthetic food additives. I recommend the use of salt in moderation, but to avoid iodized table salt. Table salt is a well-known toxin. People with high blood pressure know to avoid table salt. You don't have to wait to get high blood pressure to stop eating it; it's not good for you. Table salt has added chemicals that do not belong in your body. I want you to choose quality salt. Ask yourself, what kind of salt would a profit-based fast food chain give out for free? You may say, "But it's *fortified with* iodine, doesn't that make it good for you?" When you see the word *fortified with* exchange it with *marketed with*. You have to realize that these companies are businesses. The only reason they would add anything to their product that increases cost and lowers profit is…MARKETING.

When using salt for cooking, choose a high-quality Celtic sea salt or Himalayan salt. Our bodies accumulate toxins from foods and the environment. Foods that are dried or dehydrated can have increased concentrations of toxins and pesticides. So, minimize the use of processed condiments. When available choose organic herbs and spices for your foods.

Just because a product is sold to the public does not make it safe for your Nervous System. Nearly every restaurant in America places little packets of synthetic poisons (artificial sweeteners) on the table. Some of these artificial sweeteners even state on their packaging that their product produces tumors in lab animals. People don't seem to take these cautions seriously. There was a time in my life when I didn't either. I do now because I changed my focus away from the newest sitcom, celebrity breakdown and sensational news story to focusing my attention on making loving, healthier choices about how I invest my time, and loving myself, my family and others. I share this information with you because you and your family deserve to understand the foundations of health. Just as I stop my child from putting something harmful into her body, I am telling you to be cautious of what you allow into your mind and body.

My big realization came when I learned clinical nutrition and recognized that *everything* I had been taught about health and nutrition had been through a marketing campaign. We have a profit-based education system. By providing grants and other financial means to teachers and book authors, companies proliferate only the knowledge that benefits the company. In the medical profession, most authors and schools are funded by chemical and pharmaceutical drug companies. The research grants are primarily funded by these same companies. Medical and professional journals are sponsored through advertising from these companies. These companies control the public's knowledge of "health" and use this knowledge as a marketing tool from sitcoms to children's toys. I could go on but the bottom line is that I was sick and fat, and I wanted the most amazing life and health possible. I realized that I had to reevaluate all the knowledge I gained through food marketing, television programming and my professional education. I'm still breaking patterns today by asking myself, "Does this expand my Nervous System? Does this collapse my Nervous System?" Within a two-year period, I stopped watching media-based television, and I started integrating my Nervous System into my surroundings through physical fitness and intense research. I went from the unhealthiest I've ever been in my life to recovering the health of my youth. Once you recognize how to evaluate yourself through your Nervous System, you can guide your reality experience toward your wildest dreams.

Synthetic Chemicals Do Not Belong in the Body!

Most things labeled as nutrition are synthetic forms of vitamins. There are low fat phudes, plastic margarines and a colorful assortment of synthetic phude additives on most tables in the world. Your quality of life depends on the basic understanding that these things are not real; they are *phoney phudes*. They do not sustain or support your Nervous System. You should be able to look at any list of ingredients and recognize immediately if it contains real food or if it is a synthetic-based product. The exact ingredients don't matter. The important point is if they are synthetic. Anything labeled "artificial" *anything* (flavors, sweeteners, colors, fragrances), or if it has a chemical name, is synthetic. If it is synthetic or genetically modified, it does not belong in your body!

II. The Dangers of GMO

If you want to get healthy and live a Nervous System conscious life, you must have a strong understanding of food. Food is being manipulated in the lab much like the legend of Frankenstein but on a cellular level. A genetically modified organism (*GM* or *GMO*, also called "genetically engineered") is a microorganism (e.g., virus, bacterium) that is created in a lab to overcome natural processes. Genetic engineering involves crossing species which could not cross in nature. For example, genes from fish have been inserted into strawberries and tomatoes.

The Food and Drug Administration officially insists that *"the agency is not aware of any information showing that foods derived by these new methods differ from other foods in any meaningful or uniform way"* (FDA Statement of policy May 29, 1992). This policy was stated even after the FDA's own scientists reported that GM crops may concentrate toxins, such as heavy metals and herbicides, from the environment. The toxins in GM [livestock] feed might concentrate into milk or meat (Genetic Roulette, page 150-151).

The American Academy of Environmental Medicine, in 2009, suggested that *every doctor should place every patient on a non-GM diet*. The animal feeding studies referenced in this review tell it all. Mice that were fed GM corn had fewer babies with lower birth weights. Mice fed GM soy had testicular abnormalities and damaged sperm cells. DNA abnormalities were also found in their babies. In pregnant lab rats that were fed GM soy, 50 percent of their babies died within three weeks of being born, as compared to only ten percent of those eating non-GM soy.

This is a global public health pandemic. Most corn on the planet is genetically modified. The modified corn is registered as a pesticide because the corn itself produces BT (*Bacillus thuringiensis*) pesticides. BT, when naturally occurring, is a bacterium that attacks insects. This bacterium is considered to be safe and beneficial as a natural pest control. This is not the case once it has been genetically modified.

As novel as the idea of designing corn to create its own pesticide may be, we have to consider the effects beyond its convenience. We must ask serious questions about introducing synthetic phudes into our food supply. Does it stop producing pesticide once it has been consumed? Industry advocates claim that these pesticide-producing microbes do not survive the digestion process.

In the only human feeding trial ever published, it was confirmed that genetic material from Roundup Ready® Soybeans was transferred into the gut bacteria in three of its seven human volunteers (Genetic Roulette, pages 128-131). The GM bacteria were assimilated into their bodies, and became part of the intestinal flora of their digestive tract. Other studies have demonstrated that these bacteria may live in the body for long periods of time. In other words, these people were producing some measurable amount of BT pesticide in their guts, possibly for the rest of their lives.

Many animals have a sixth sense that allows them to recognize the difference between GM phudes and real food. When given a side-by-side choice, animals will choose to eat the real foods. Humans don't seem to have that same ability. The population is unaware that genetically modified phudes even exist much less that they are on the dinner table. Most of the public's palate has been destroyed by the ingestion of synthetic phudes and chemical additives. Their palates have been burned by these chemicals making their taste buds dull. People who eat fast phudes need a lot of salt, spices, condiments and flavor enhancers to make their phude taste good. When a person has a clean diet, their palate won't tolerate the taste of the synthetic chemicals commonly used in fast phudes. When you have a clean palate, you taste the actual flavors of the food.

- There are four ways to avoid GM products:

- Buy organic

- Buy products labeled non-GM or non-GMO

- Buy products listed on the non-GMO shopping guide found on www.ResponsibleTechnology.org. Avoid high risk GM ingredients: alfalfa , canola, corn, cottonseed, soy and sugar

Europeans Don't Have To Eat GM *Phudes*, So Why Do We?

In April 1999, the people of Europe stood up against the GM phude industry. Within one week, all the major food suppliers removed GM ingredients from their products. Today in America, the only way to easily get non-GM fed cheese and meats is to buy those imported from Europe. The same food producers that removed GM ingredients from their food products in Europe continue to feed GM ingredients to Americans.

Genetically engineered bovine growth hormone (rBGH) was removed from Walmarts and other major U.S. food chains in 2006. It takes relatively few people to shift retailers from using harmful products. It only takes about five percent of the population to create awareness large enough to shift a retailer's supply chain. We have to raise our voices about choosing real foods over GM phudes. If you take one thing from this book, let it be to avoid purchasing or consuming GM phudes. Please research this and tell everyone you know to stop eating GM phudes. Their life and health depend on it!

Avoid Irradiated Foods

Governments around the world are being lobbied by the food and pharmaceutical industries to irradiate all our food. Irradiation greatly increases the shelf life of a product by killing off any living DNA, good or bad, within the food. The enzymes within food aid digestion of that same food. A banana will keep quite a while on the shelf. But, once nature's seal is broken and the peel is cracked, within minutes, the yellow flesh of the banana begins to turn brown. The enzymes within the food begin to rapidly digest the fruit.

Killing the enzymes may be great for a store that wants to sell you old apples, but what does that do to you and your health? First of all, those enzymes transfer the nutrients to your body. The body uses the enzymes within the fruit for its digestion. The damage to these enzymes caused by irradiation will decrease the body's ability to absorb the nutrients. Ionizing radiation can have a cumulative effect on your body. I am concerned that each bite of food containing radiation can bioaccumulate over time. Even if your body could process this radiation, the energy necessary to process this toxic energy field can contribute to neurological collapse. The public is not aware this is even an issue. Most people are not aware of the health concerns posed by genetically modified or irradiated food. They are not aware of which foods on the shelf are genetically modified because there is no requirement to label GM foods. The FDA has claimed that there is no difference and, therefore, no need to label the difference between genetically modified phudes and organic foods.

When the population recognizes that government systems have allowed laws to be selfishly written and lobbied by the chemical and food industries to benefit the industries themselves and not the public, it starts making more sense. The FDA has been infiltrated by industry insiders and allowed products and technology to be released into the public that have not been adequately tested and cannot be recalled. They are allowing genetic pollution into the food supply and into our bodies.

The rules are no longer there to protect us; instead, the rules now ensure we get the minimum nutrition and care necessary to sustain life. Are you feeling it yet? These agencies have manipulated our food supply.

There are even laws that have been passed that make it illegal for you to grow your own foods, herbs and medicinal plants. Even if you have never planted a seed in your life, don't you feel you should have the right to plant a garden? Grow some fruit trees and plants such as potato, beans, lettuce, tomatoes or herbs, such as oregano, basil and mint? Cultivate for yourself the healthiest nutrient dense food on the planet for soil, water and time? If we cannot grow our own food, we are forced to buy minimum-standard genetically modified crap phudes. When the food supply is manipulated, it hinders the body's ability to regenerate, protect, project and heal itself. There are no synthetic replacements for real food.

We are seeing malnourishment, toxic symptoms and illnesses manifest in a well-fed population. The well-fed population is malnourished because they are eating phony phudes. There are few, if any, useful nutrients in phoney phudes. These phudes should be considered toxins because, rather than giving us energy, it takes us physical energy to process them.

In addition to being harmful for our bodies, these phoney phudes are also bad for the environment, because they alter the DNA of the food chain. These toxin-producing living organisms are in corn. We are eating foods containing living organisms that produce toxins even insects won't eat. If bugs, bacteria and animals will not eat a plant, it is not fit for human consumption.

Avoid GM: Alfalfa, Canola, Corn, Cottonseed, Soy and Sugar

The main genetically modified foods to look out for are alfalfa, canola, corn, cottonseed, soy, and sugar from sugar beets. Corn has been so affected that it is nearly impossible to find corn that is not genetically modified. I am Mexican, and a huge part of my heritage is based on eating corn, which is now unsafe for us to eat.

I did not understand the seriousness of this issue until I watched the documentary film *World According to Monsanto*. The destruction of the world's corn supply is devastating. I highly suggest that you watch this movie with your family and children. If I risk eating corn, it must be labeled organic. Otherwise I recommend that you teach your young ones that "corn has chemicals" and should be avoided.

It is especially hard to avoid corn during the holidays. In my culture, it is customary to have corn tortillas, tamales and countless other traditional foods made with corn. These food traditions have been poisoned by genetically modified phudes. It is scary to see my culture, my heritage, being destroyed through phudes. It is truly disgusting to watch it happen, and to see young children suffering from severe obesity, diabetes, neurological disorders and chronic illnesses. It breaks my heart to have to tell my daughter that we don't eat corn, because it has chemicals. Parents unknowingly feed their children phony phudes that look and taste like foods that they have lived on for generations. Not everyone can digest or physically process phony phude. The people who cannot will suffer from chronic illness and obesity.

High Fructose Corn Syrup Made with Mercury

The *Environmental Health Journal* published an article stating that the average American consumes up to 28 micrograms of mercury per day in foods containing *high fructose corn syrup* (HFCS). High fructose corn syrup is the genetically modified sweetener found in almost everything packaged. Check the ingredients before you eat anything. Ingredients are labeled in order by weight. The most prevalent ingredient in the product will be listed first, the second most prevalent is second, and so on. HFCS is usually listed in the top three ingredients of most packaged products. Search: "high fructose corn syrup aliases" to find a list of ingredients that are "also known as" or "partially made from" high fructose corn syrup. The bottom line is: if it's processed and packaged, it likely has high fructose corn syrup. HFCS, with or without mercury, does not support or sustain your Nervous System and does not belong in your body.

We cannot leave our nutrition and health to be dictated by what is most profitable for the phude and chemical industries. We must retain our health freedom. Our lives depend on it. A new model for health must be designed around the health needs of each individual's Nervous System. If you have followed television's version of health, as I did for many years, you are likely on the road to obesity, chronic illness and early death.

III.   Real Immunity

> *"When the Nervous System is strengthened,*
> *the body will heal itself."*
> —George Gonzalez, DC, QN

Real immunity begins with a non-GM nourished mother breast-feeding her child. Breast milk is the most amazing food source on the planet. Its chemical makeup changes moment to moment depending on the child's needs. This nourishing liquid is alive; it has intelligence. It supports the Nervous System through exponential physical and nonphysical growth and development. It demonstrates amazing healing properties and is the only food made for the developing human Nervous System.

Thankfully, at this time, it is not illegal to breast feed your child. But a word of caution: the formula industry nearly wiped out the use of breast-feeding. They somehow managed to convince the world that their convenient, mercury-laden high fructose corn syrup made with tap water, fortified with chlorine and fluoride is better than breast milk. In the future, the negative campaign against feeding your child raw breast milk may be based on the reasons that are now making raw dairy illegal to purchase.

As breast milk is unpasteurized, not radiated and it has not been fortified with vitamins and minerals to ensure the minimum daily allowance, its nutrients cannot be measured to guarantee consistency. The amount of breast milk consumed cannot be measured, so there's no way of knowing if the child is getting adequate nutrition. There may be a "tittie tax" to fund the bureaucracy around the right to feed your child naturally.

Believe it or not, elements of the "right" to breastfeed have been fought in the highest court in the United States. Thankfully, breast-feeding has been found to be a constitutional right. But I want to emphasize that it was challenged. We had to fight for it! What if the right had been lost? What if it had just slipped away without anyone noticing? Children have managed to survive for thousands of years and thrive on breast milk. Why would feeding your child ever become a crime? Because it doesn't make the phude industries any money!

Human Breast Milk Is the Only Food on the Planet Uniquely Designed and Formulated to Feed the Human Nervous System.

There are many benefits to breast-feeding. Those that stand out include that it reduces breast cancer in the women who breastfeed. Children that are breastfed have a higher IQ and it naturally decreases their chances of diabetes, cancer and obesity. As any lactation consultant will tell you, breast milk has amazing healing properties. Breast milk is "liquid" Nervous System. It can be used over cuts and wounds for accelerated healing. I mostly avoid dairy because a cow's milk is ideal for the development of a cow's Nervous System. A cow's nutrient needs are different from a human's. We are the only animal on the planet that completely nourishes our children with the milk of another species.

Real Foods in Their Most Natural Form

The raw food movement presents a strong philosophy based in feeding the body organic, nutrient-dense, living foods. This philosophy presents a strong model for healing the body with food. For free videos online, search: "healing with raw foods." I have trained many people how to reverse their disease process by eating and using raw foods. When you properly feed the Nervous System, the functions become efficient. Freed energy is now focused on detoxifying and healing the body. We should focus on providing the body with the purest, most nutrient dense foods available.

Juicing for Rapid Healing

I have found that juicing your vegetables is a great way to pack the nutrient dense foods into your body necessary for rapid healing. I only juice non-GM fruits and vegetables, preferably organic. Apple, carrot and beet juice are wonderful, but I only recommend them in small quantities. I only use them to sweeten the bitterness of the most efficient Nervous System fuel—dark, leafy green vegetables. I use the most nutrient-dense dark greens available: spinach, kale, romaine and celery. I juice them all together and use as little apple, carrot or beet juice necessary to sweeten it to taste.

The more health compromised a person is, the less apple, carrot and beet juice should be used. More serious conditions and infections can thrive on sugar fed by the sweet juice. "Going raw," or, becoming a person who primarily eats raw foods, can be a bit of a culture shock. You would think that not cooking food makes it easier to feed yourself. I experienced relearning how to prepare and eat foods in their natural state and how to combine natural flavors to satisfy my palate. This can be difficult to do 100 percent of the time, yet the closer I can get my diet to 100 percent raw, the better I feel.

Packaged raw foods are great alternatives to packaged commercial foods. Snacks and treats made from raw, vegan, gluten-free, non-GM foods are incredible. People can over eat packaged, raw food just as they over eat synthetic phudes. Raw foods are not guilt-free, but without the synthetic chemical burden, your body can process raw packaged foods more easily by comparison.

My suggestion is to focus on eating foods in their natural state. When you increase the raw foods you eat, it is easy to only eat the fruits and vegetables you currently enjoy. So, I urge you to explore new foods and discover real flavors. There are plenty of free videos online that teach you how to prepare raw food in simple and delicious ways.

Going raw is a process. Few people can live the lifestyle 100 percent of the time. Incrementally increase the percentage of raw foods you are eating. Think of transitioning into a way of eating, as opposed to dramatically altering the way you eat 100 percent by tomorrow morning.

Cooking Foods Damages Vital Nutrients and Enzymes

Cooking your foods over 120° F will begin to kill the enzymes and nutrients within the food. Microwave (radiation) destroys all life within the food completely. I avoid food or water cooked in a microwave.

Dr. Royal Lee, dentist and founder of Standard Process, Inc., a clinical nutrition company, makes products from raw food ingredients. He was very concerned with the health effects caused by eating processed foods and wanted to offset the free radical damage. His preference for ideal health was primarily a raw food diet with occasional dairy and lean organ and muscle meats. He suggested that, to offset the free radical damage caused by cooking the food, we should eat an equal amount of raw foods: 50 percent cooked food and 50 percent raw food.

This recommendation was first given back in the 1930s when food was still naturally organic but simple, synthetic phude processing was becoming more common. It was at this time the dental community witnessed instances where their patients' teeth inexplicably began to rot in their heads. The common threads in all the cases were their patients' diets. As consumption of *foods of commerce* (processed foods) increased, the population became malnourished, even though they were well fed with processed phudes. Dr. Lee and other doctors found that food processing strips foods of all their vital nutrients. These processed phudes were then being fortified (*marketed with*) with synthetic vitamins and minerals. He described this as similar to somebody robbing the jewels from our food supply and replacing them with glass.

Dr. Lee and other pioneers of this time warned us of damage to the food supply in the 1930's. Today we see a global scale production of synthetic foods. Today's foods have a fraction of the nutrients organic foods had before food was processed. Due to conventional farming methods, our topsoil has been depleted of its nutrients. It takes over 30 of today's apples to provide the same nutrient density of one apple from the 1800's. Given today's environment, I feel Dr. Lee's recommendation needs to be updated (and I feel he would agree). I am suggesting that, to offset the damage from today's cooked foods, we triple the portion of raw fruits and vegetables to 25 percent cooked foods and 75 percent raw fruits and vegetables. I also recommend a gluten-free diet and avoiding all wheat and grain products. I personally do my best to avoid all corns and grains, including rice. The varieties of these grains available today tend to cause inflammation that can aggravate and contribute to chronic illness.

IV. What is Clean?

The common illusion of clean is poisonous and deadly. Just pick up any cleaning product to read the back panel and you will often find: "harmful if swallowed," "eye hazard," "call poison control," "keep out of reach of children." Do you think these products are safe for our Nervous Systems? These chemicals may kill germs, but they add to our synthetic burden that can cause or contribute to chronic illness and death.

What Does Not Kill the Bacteria Makes it Stronger

The discovery of penicillin and antibiotics has changed our lives. Although they have been gifts to humanity, they have done so at the expense of the body's natural ecosystem. These life-saving drugs can often destroy the good bacteria in the digestive tract allowing yeast and fungus to overtake the body and potentially causing chronic illness. Most people have difficulty with their digestion after a round of antibiotics, making them more susceptible to developing irritable bowel syndrome, yeast infections, sexual dysfunction and malnutrition.

The bacteria within our bodies that are exposed to antibiotics and survive will develop a resistance to that particular antibiotic. Once the bacteria in a person's body have developed a resistance to an antibiotic, the person will have to resort to using a different antibiotic. After a few rounds of the new antibiotic, the bacteria in the body eventually become resistant to the second antibiotic, as well. Once exposed and resistant to multiple antibiotics, these infections are called MRSA (Methicillin-resistant *Staphylococcus aureus*, pronounced "Mersa"). MRSA refers to bacteria that can no longer be managed with antibiotics. The only way to fight off these types of infections is by strengthening the Nervous System to fend for itself.

Avoid Antibiotics and Antibacterial Products

The over use of prescription antibiotics and antibacterial products in daily life exposes more and more bacteria to different antibiotics. My personal strategy is to use antibiotics as little as possible. I do my best to heal my body without resorting to them. I feed my body the most nutritious food and nutrients available to support my body's ability to fight off disease and infection naturally. Because the day that I need antibiotics—in a life or death situation—I want them to work. I don't want my body's ecosystem to have been prematurely overexposed to the antibiotics that may one day save my life.

We have been trained in what it means to be "clean" and how to "clean" by the chemical industry. In reality, harsh detergents, chemicals and antibiotics strip dirt and germs away leaving an ecosystem permanently destroyed and vulnerable to future infection. We have to redefine how things are cleaned. Using toxic chemicals to clean anything destroys all life and, therefore, will not sustain yours.

Our Daily Synthetic Burden

Using chemicals in your daily life adds to your synthetic burden. The world is under an illusion that the only way to clean things is by adding toxic chemicals. I find it far superior to clean things using products with natural enzymes and essential oils with other naturally occurring ingredients. Using these products will naturally clean your environment without making it toxic.

The synthetic chemical industry has lied to us and created synthetic products to clean, freshen and disinfect. These synthetic chemicals are not good for our bodies. I'm not saying that we shouldn't clean things. I am saying we should clean things without synthetic chemicals and antibiotics in them.

Our synthetic chemical burden is best managed at home. But caution must be taken not to use or bring synthetics into your home. The products used to wash your clothes, floors, kitchen, pans, plates and utensils can also add to your toxic burden. Body care products can be loaded with synthetic chemicals. If you do not have a water filter on your shower or home, you are breathing in noxious chlorine and fluoride fumes, as well as absorbing them through your skin. Hazardous chemicals, such as mineral oils, sodium lauryl sulfates, lye, ammonia, formaldehyde, kerosene, phenol, sulfuric acid, sulfamic acid, among others, are commonly used in skin care lotions, suntan oils and body washes. All these chemicals are absorbed by your skin and can *off gas* (release toxic odors) throughout the day.

You may be surprised to know that even your clothing can be toxic. To my knowledge, there is no regulation on chemicals used to color or process clothing. The detergents used for washing clothing can also be toxic. For a chemically sensitive person like me, walking down the detergent aisle in the supermarket is a test of how long I can hold my breath. Smelling chemical detergents and fabric softener on washed clothing can initiate an allergic response, breathing problems and headaches. If it can make me sick within seconds, what is it doing to the person wearing these clothes all day long? Even if he or she is not as sensitive as I am, it's necessary to process the synthetic burden of these chemicals. The body still absorbs these chemicals through the skin and in every breath. I recommend using fragrance free products, using less detergent or double rinsing your clothes until there is no odor from the detergent.

Cooking at home is often considered to be a healthier alternative to eating out. There are, however, pitfalls to be avoided here, too. Healthy eating begins with non-GM foods. Many people wash their fruits and vegetables in the sink using unfiltered water. Our foods absorb the chlorine and other chemicals in the tap water as they're being washed. Cooking on nonstick pans releases fluoride fumes into your food from the nonstick surfaces. Most vegetable oils and sprays are made of GM ingredients. Margarine is a synthetic phude. You can think of it as a plasticized fat. The table salt is loaded with chemicals and fortified (marketed with) iodine. Most condiments used in the United States, such as ketchup, mustard, mayonnaise and teriyaki sauce, among others, are made of GM ingredients and contain mercury from high fructose corn syrup. Seasonings and sauces can contain toxic pesticides and chemicals such as MSG (monosodium glutamate). This flavor enhancer is a known toxin causing severe allergies, migraines, digestive distress and even death.

Unfortunately, eating out makes it more difficult to manage our synthetic burden. At least, when you are at home, you have personal control and can remove the synthetics mentioned above from your lifestyle. It's far worse when you leave your home, because you have little or no control over the products used by the establishments you visit. The detergents used to clean the restaurant are likely toxic. I don't like putting my bare arms on a table top freshly sprayed with chemicals. I also won't let my child eat food that has fallen onto the tabletop of the restaurant. In addition to avoiding the cleaning chemicals used in restaurants, I recommend avoiding the high risk GM ingredients: alfalfa, canola, corn, cottonseed, soy and sugar. If you're eating in a restaurant and your meal is made of one of these ingredients, it is likely you are eating GM phudes.

I could keep describing every facet of your life, but I think you understand my point. We have to minimize the toxic burden on our bodies. In my opinion, the only way to do that is to completely remove synthetics from our bodies and our foods. This means surrounding ourselves with products made from natural, renewable sources. Your body care should be edible and organic. Do your best to avoid all known synthetics. It is impossible to avoid them completely in our modern society, but if we can do our best to keep synthetics out of our daily lives, out of our homes, out of our foods, and out of our bodies, we will remove a significant portion of the toxic chemical burden from our Nervous Systems.

Chapter 7

KEY #5: THE BODY HEALS ITSELF

"The power that made the body, heals the body!"
—B.J. Palmer, DC Pioneer of Chiropractic

In order to explore Nervous System Consciousness, we must explore the boundaries of our Nervous System. We have discovered a new frontier in Nervous System communication. We must allow the Nervous System's intelligence to guide the body's healing.

Our Nervous System communication can be broken down into two major areas: physical and nonphysical. *Physical* communication includes all communication activity which occurs within the body (internal) and that which occurs outside of the body received through our five senses (external). *Nonphysical* (holographic) communication considers many aspects of communication between cells, self, others, the universe and our spiritual connection.

Physical and Internal Environment

The *internal* environment considers all the communication which occurs within your physical body. It includes the body's physical movement and the logistics and transfer of physical units within the body. A long list of cellular communication, neurotransmitters, hormones, insulin, pH, blood chemistry, blood pressure, oxygen levels and anything else that can be measured physically and occurs within the physical frame of the body is placed in this physical communication environment.

To appreciate the communication available within the physical environment, we can focus on the cell. Every cell of the body has over one million receptors. We do not have full knowledge of every receptor on every cell of the body. Considering the trillions of cells, each with millions of receptors, that's a lot of terrain that we know absolutely nothing about. Entire industries are dedicated to studying the actions that occur within cells.

The medical industry has placed most of its focus on the center of the cell, the DNA. The biotechnology, pharmaceutical and nano-technology industries have spent billions if not trillions of dollars and countless lifetimes of man-hours on studying cells. The strides we have made in understanding the cell and its functions and communications are incredible. In that amazement of our technological advancement, this knowledge is rudimentary in comparison to that of your existing Nervous System. The shock is we know very little about cellular communication and technology.

Cellular and Nervous System life forms, such as amoebas, animals and humans, have been on this planet for unknown centuries without our current medical and scientific contributions. The amazing intelligence that made your body was already here and works without your mental contribution. Your body can heal itself without your understanding of how it heals.

In Quantum Neurology®, we use the Nervous System's intelligence to guide the healing process. Corrections are only made if they demonstrate neurological benefit. We trust the intelligence of the Nervous System to guide its own rehabilitation because *the power that made the body heals the body!"*

Physical and External Environment

Our Nervous System also communicates with a second area that I referred to as the *external* environment. This includes all connections of the Nervous System to our physical surroundings, which extend into the universe. We record the experiences of our physical surroundings with our five senses (sight, hearing, smell, taste and touch). Damage, delay or loss in any of our five senses can be devastating. Our quality of life depends on our Nervous System's ability to receive and process information from the external environment instantaneously.

Nonphysical (Holographic) Environment

The third area of Nervous System communication is *nonphysical (holographic)*. The mind, thoughts, emotions and spiritual connection are examples of the communication occurring in the nonphysical environment. This environment is not limited by space, time or location. Because it is not physical, it exists everywhere and nowhere simultaneously. It just simply is.

The Nervous System also controls entry of nonphysical information and thought. Physically, we can block sound by covering our ears. But on an unconscious level, the same pattern is evident in the way most people have difficulty thinking of life without a close friend, family member or themselves. We see this with people who avoid talking about life insurance or planning for the family after the death of a spouse. When the subject comes up they may say, "I can't go there." A third example may be someone who is in denial and not able or willing to see a situation from a different perspective, such as an addict unable to see or acknowledge how the drug of choice is damaging his or her life.

There is an invisible force field which contains your essence, thoughts and emotions connected to your physical body. These invisible fields of holographic communication control the parameters of the entire Nervous System. We can explain the communication environment of the Nervous System separately, but, just as the systems of the body function in tandem, it all works in perfect unison.

Focused Intention

When I changed my focus toward cultivating and expanding my Nervous System, it completely changed my life. In order to be better at anything in life, it must be accomplished through the Nervous System.

I began to look at my life: career, finances, relationships, spirituality and family. I evaluated where I was in each area. Then, I dreamed of what was possible. I saw how my dreams directed my LightBody projection, and my life began to occupy the space created by the light projected from my dreams. As simple as that sounds, it was truly a profound change.

The Yawn Field

As a fish does not know it lives in water, we do not know we live in light. We are so connected that we lose sight of how we are all connected in light consciousness. The yawn field is a perfect example of this invisible connection we all share.

Do you know what it's like to catch a yawn? You see someone yawns, then you yawn and—even if you just talk about the yawn...we all start yawning. We have all caught a yawn. As a public speaker, if I yawn in front of the group, I can watch the audience begin to yawn like popcorn. Most people yawn in their own time, some in unison.

I call this the yawn field because it is a connection we all share. When we look at yawning, it displays attributes of nonphysical communication. It defies time, space and location. If you were to watch a video of someone yawning, you could catch the yawn. It does not matter whether the video was recorded a moment earlier or years before. This concept is not limited to video initiated yawns. In fact, I am yawning as I write this, and I am sure you are having a hard time reading this without yawning.

Get a Yawn

Some people have difficulty relaxing and initiating sleep. Their body is so stuck in the *sympathetic* fight and flight actions of the Nervous System that their body can't shift down into the rest, digest and heal actions of the *parasympathetic* Nervous System. Try using this when you are having trouble relaxing or going to sleep. Retract your jaw by using your jaw muscles to pull your chin back toward your head. Then, look at a light or something bright and take a slow, deep breath while blinking your eyes. This should initiate a yawn indicating a shift towards the *parasympathetic* Nervous System.

This is just one example of how the body's natural actions, reactions and reflexes can be used to shift the Nervous System towards a desired activity naturally.

Autonomic Reactions

Autonomic reactions are the Nervous System's actions that are not controlled by intellect; they are automatic. Examples of *autonomic reactions* are yawning, sighing, laughing, sneezing, burping, sweating and chills down your spine or body, to name a few. The Nervous System discharges stress from the nonphysical environment through autonomic reactions.

Continuing with yawning as an example of a Nervous System discharge, we yawn when we are sleepy and bored. We yawn when we see others yawning. We also share this odd connection with all mammals. Watch any nature show and notice that you will yawn when other animals yawn. I feel that a yawn is a physical action that discharges nonphysical stress. It is the pressure release valve for the Nervous System's nonphysical aspects. Like burping the lid of a plastic container to expel excess air, yawning (and all other autonomic reactions) discharges stress from your Nervous System.

Autonomic Reactions in Healing

Healing happens automatically with or without your mental contribution. The yawn field demonstrates the autonomic field of the body. We have found clinically that when we tap in to the healing attributes of the Nervous System, we set off autonomic reactions. This discharge occurs in the person who's Nervous System is most able to release it. We have to remember this is not initiated physically; it is initiated through the nonphysical.

When we perform Nervous System rehabilitation on a patient, the yawn field demonstrates in anyone associated with the patient. This includes the doctor, patient and anyone emotionally connected to the patient or anyone watching the session live or recorded. This phenomenon also occurs when we talk or think about a person. If the patient's session is on video, any person watching the tape in the future will demonstrate autonomic reactions just as watching a comedy makes you laugh (autonomic reaction) every time you watch it even when you know the punch line.

I personally have an autonomic twitch that occurs when I perform Nervous System rehabilitation on someone. I can feel energy build up in my body, and, when it discharges, my head shakes. I also experience other autonomic discharges through respiration changes, sighing and bursts of sweat, among many others. I use these autonomic discharges as an indicator that I am working within the holographic field of the Nervous System. Although people may find it amusing to watch my head twitch when I discharge autonomic stress while working on someone, it is *not* something that I can control. People often ask what it feels like, and I often respond by saying, "What does sneezing feel like?" I feel a sensation of energy building up within my body. It's much like sneezing or yawning. The wave of energy builds and then... "Ahhh-chooo!" You can observe the actions with your own body. The autonomic healing reactions feel similar to the buildup of a sneeze or a yawn.

Healing Detox Reactions

In order to get healthy from any injury, infection, illness or condition, the Nervous System needs to clear the battlefield and rebuild. Much like de-cluttering a room, the Nervous System needs to release the toxins and cellular debris from their storage sites and transport them out of the Nervous System. During the body's removal of cellular debris and toxins, the body may experience a flare up of symptoms. These flare ups can be serious if the person's body is releasing toxins faster than they can be flushed out. This is referred to as a *Herxheimer (Herx) reaction* or healing reaction.

Detoxification is a sign the Nervous System is healing. We want to see this when working with patients, because this means the body is mobilizing toxins to discharge them from the Nervous System. Compare that to a Nervous System that does not kick up its dust to clean house. When the Nervous System is in collapse, it fails to reach toward self-healing. It does not have the resources to kick up the dust to clean house. Our challenge is to remove the debris and synthetic burden from the Nervous System, while maintaining its open channels of elimination, to avoid a strong healing reaction.

Hydration

Our body is primarily made of water, and we need to maintain proper fluid intake to hydrate every cell of our body. A person can only live from two days to a week without water, depending on the circumstances. Toxins and cellular debris must be flushed regularly from your body with good clean spring or filtered water. Be cautious of tap water because many areas of the world add toxic chemicals to the water supply. Search: "drugs found in tap water." Chlorine, fluoride, lithium, lye and pharmaceutical medications are chemicals commonly used. These synthetic chemicals do not belong in your body and cause untold damage to the environment and our ecosystem. Investigate the water source from your area. Where does your tap water come from? How is the pH of your water stabilized? Is it recycled sewage water? How is it being filtered?

When you think about how vital water is to your survival, it's important to know everything about where our water comes from. Professionally, I educate people to drink half of their body weight in ounces of water per day. For example: A 100 pound person should drink 50 ounces of water per day. (50 ounces is approximately 1.5 liter.)

Water is Alive

There are many traditions that use water to carry holy, healing or energetic qualities. Homeopathy uses dilutions of toxins in water. The toxin is so diluted that only the memory, or vibration, of the toxin remains. The diluted toxin can initiate a healing reaction within the body. Water exhibits consciousness and memory. Your body's hydration contributes to your body's ability to project and access the consciousness and memory of your LightBody.

Dr. Masaru Emoto of Japan has documented the effect of intent on water. Taking samples of water from distilled, natural springs and lakes, glaciers, and holy water sources, Dr. Emoto froze samples from each source and examined their crystalline structure under a dark field microscope. Then, he exposed the water samples to various stimuli, including music, prayers from religious leaders, loving or hurtful chants, hand written messages ranging from love to hatred, written in ink on the exterior of water bottles. The effect of the stimulus on the water was amazing. The frozen water's crystalline structure took on a shape generated by the intention of the stimulus. Symmetry and beauty appeared when the water was subjected to words reflecting praise and honor. The crystalline structures derived from the same water sources, when exposed to messages of hatred and ugliness, projected an obvious difference. Their dingy color and lack of shape and symmetry reflected the malintent.

This work demonstrates the power of intention. The water samples in Dr. Emoto's research demonstrated water's affinity for good intention by its shape and symmetry. Intention allows the water to express its maximum projection. Our bodies are made primarily of water. When we realize that every thought and every word contributes to the water's projection, we must, then, realize that every thought and every word contributes to our Nervous System's projection, as well.

Filter Your Water

Clean water is necessary to sustain life. Only one percent of the water on earth is fit for human consumption. To thrive in today's society water filtration is a must! It is difficult to survive without using tap water, so consider filtering the water that comes into your home. Ideally, you could filter the water in the entire home. Otherwise, each home should have a minimum of two filters: a shower filter to minimize your exposure to chemicals when showering, and a counter top water filter or a jug with a replaceable filter in your kitchen. Wash all your food in filtered water. Wear gloves when you are handling unfiltered city water. Use non-toxic soap to clean your dishes. You do not want to consume any of these chemicals that may remain on your dishes after washing. Using natural cleaning supplies will also minimize the synthetic burden on the future water supply.

pH: Power of Hydrogen

To have a healthy and conscious life you must have a chemically balanced Nervous System. Your pH is a measurement of your body's acid or alkaline level. It can be monitored at home by a simple and inexpensive saliva or urine test. You body pH will be most affected and can be managed with the foods you eat.

PH stands for powers of hydrogen (or potential hydrogen) and is the unit used to measure the acid/alkaline levels of liquids. Our bodies function best within a certain range of acid/alkaline balance.

PH is measured in a range from: 0-14 where zero is the most acidic and 14 is the most alkaline (basic). Stomach acid should have a pH of 1, distilled water has a pH of 7 and bleach has a pH of 13. Our bodies are 90 percent water, so our natural pH balance within our body occurs within the 6 to 8 range. Urinary pH should be between 6 to 7. Ideal salivary pH should be 7.2. Most health food stores will sell pH paper that you can use to test yourself daily. When your body is in proper balance, your biochemistry is working within the ideal range.

When the body is either too acidic or too alkaline, the body is outside of this ideal range and chemical processes are altered or delayed. In dentistry, when your salivary pH shifts, your mouth, teeth and gums become vulnerable to infection and cavities. Your teeth are important indicators of your health. The sudden onset of cavities caused by acidic saliva indicates a significant health shift. Gout and other arthritic conditions are also caused by a buildup in acid levels within the body.

The bottom line to balancing and maintaining your pH naturally is by eating green vegetables (preferably raw). Romaine, kale, spinach, chard and celery are a few great examples. These vegetables are so important because they provide a protective chemical barrier from the acids that cause damage in your body. This is called a *"buffer."* The buildup of a buffer in your body is crucial for managing pH. Consider it money in your health account that prevents disease and helps your body manage its biochemistry.

Entire healing strategies, philosophies and lifestyles are built around balancing pH. One example is the macrobiotic philosophy of eating which focuses on the selection and preparation of foods that create an ideal pH balance for your body. Emphasized is chewing food until it is liquid before swallowing to ensure that the digestive enzymes in saliva saturate the food you eat. This philosophy and lifestyle is attributed to curing many people of chronic and degenerative diseases. The macrobiotic lifestyle is not for everyone, but we can learn from the wisdom of these healing strategies.

Your body's biochemistry begins in the mouth. As infants, our first reflex is called the suckling reflex. This reflex initiates our body's digestion through saliva. When saliva pH is 7.2, it lays the foundation for the proper chemical balance of your entire body.

Lymphatics

The lymphatic system is your body's natural detoxification system, or sewage disposal network. It picks up all the dead cells, toxins and debris from the trillions of body cells and moves them toward the heart, lungs and liver for processing out of the body. Unlike our blood circulation, which is pumped by the heart, lymphatics are *passive* and depend on your body's movement to move the toxins and debris out.

When you get sick, your lymph nodes swell because they are overburdened with sludge. You have lymph nodes all over your body, but the ones most easily recognized when you're sick are those on your neck below your jaw, under your arms and in your groin. Just as your home can get filled with clutter and garbage if you don't take the trash out for collection, your body can get filled with toxins stuck in the lymphatic channel. When you understand how lymph moves though the body, you can help it process toxins and enhance your body's natural healing process.

Here is a simple method to stimulate your body's natural detoxification. It can be done multiple times per day when you are sick and daily, for maintenance. Simply drag your fingertips on your skin toward your heart. You can drag your fingers from your ears down your neck toward your heart. You can also drag your fingers from your ankles, up the legs, toward your groin, and continue from your groin to your navel, then from your navel toward your heart. You can then use the opposite hand to drag the fingertips from the hand and wrist up the arm. Continue dragging the fingertips through the pit of the arm and toward the heart. This is performed on both sides of the body and can be repeated several times a day if necessary. This process can also be done while in the shower using the water to stimulate the lymphatics toward the heart.

Do not underestimate the healing power of removing the toxins from your body. This simple exercise can help stimulate your body to remove the physical burden of toxins, so that your body can focus on your healing instead of taking out the garbage.

Please note: Physical lymphatic stimulation is not recommended in people experiencing cancer.

Holographic Movement

Yoga, Pilates, swimming and certain martial arts demonstrate the principles of holographic movement. It is very different than the gym concept of building muscle through muscle group isolation, repetitive motions and added weight. Holographic movement focuses on using the entire Nervous System to activate function. Every cell contributes, participates or is engaged in the physical action. Swimming is an excellent example of learning to move your body as a holographic unit. As the octopus uses its amazing strength, leveraging against its own body when floating in water, we are forced to engage our entire bodies, too, when in water, and similarly when in yoga, or performing a martial art.

Walking on the treadmill may burn calories but it does not maximally engage your Nervous System. Using a treadmill isolates your Nervous System to very specific functions. It removes the need to worry about uneven ground, cars, traffic laws and other runners. I'm not telling you to go running in traffic… I'm simply saying there is a big difference in Nervous System activity between running on a treadmill and running outside.

Holographic movement embraces the principle of using every cell in your body toward a particular activity. This whole body engagement allows for holographic communication through activity. With this simple understanding, you can recognize which actions generate holographic communication, such as a simple push-up, which engages your entire body and the activities which do not, like a bicep curl. You can now customize your fitness to include or create exercises which engage every cell of your body. It won't be a surprise to find out that the people who use this concept in their fitness routines have the highest levels of fitness and the best bodies.

The Element of Danger

In addition to the concept of holographic movement, I also recommend fitness that includes the element of life and death without endangering your life. This is important because we are animals and we need to activate our "fight and flight" response. This is the *sympathetic* part of our Nervous System that is used for fighting and running away. Attributes associated to this portion of the Nervous System are strength, balance, speed and reaction time. The martial arts are a perfect example of learning to manage your Nervous System during intense situations.

Rock climbing, balancing arts and racing (in all forms) are just a few examples of activities which stimulate your fight and flight activity. This is vitally important because, in these types of activity, we develop our *sympathetic* Nervous System. Developing these activities allows for a natural and deeper transition into the "rest, digest and heal" (*parasympathetic*) actions of the Nervous System. This activity must be performed physically to discharge the nonphysical stress of the Nervous System.

Physical activity forces our bodies into a cascade of autonomic responses, including increased heart rate, respiration and sweating. Your body's ability to respond to physical stress is indicative of your Nervous System's *tone* (strength in physical and nonphysical attributes). An athlete will have a better command over managing these fight or flight responses than will non-athletes. The autonomic discharges activated during exercise allow the body to release emotional and other nonphysical stress.

When the physical activity stops, the body naturally transitions into its rest, digest and heal activities. For those that are physically able, one way to strengthen your body's healing is through exercising the physical attributes required for survival. Nervous system strength, speed, agility, balance, intelligent instantaneous action and reaction are all attributes of survival. For optimal results, physically use your Nervous System and focus on measuring and expanding all its functions.

Health is Wealth!

A holographic shift occurs when the entire Nervous System realigns its focus. This realignment will alter the LightBody projection. Using these principles within Quantum Neurology® rehabilitation, we often work with people who are disabled or crippled by their condition and restore them very quickly. People often look at me in bewilderment and ask, "How is this possible? How can you get these results when no one else has?"

We work with the Nervous System's natural actions and reflexes. We do not force the Nervous System. We use functional evaluations of strength and performance to guide the patient's care. Expansion of the Nervous System is the only indication we are interested in pursuing. The doctors that utilize these principles are stimulating natural healing to generate wellness in their patients. This includes expansion in lifestyle and fitness, proper diet, food-based nutrients, elimination and detoxification support.

The cost of health care in the United States exceeds $7,000 per person per year. This money goes into the health care industry. This money does not feed your body or train you how to get healthy.

What could you do for your health with $7,000? I, personally, would begin by affording the best foods possible—the healthiest, freshest, organically grown foods. I would only purchase body care and clothing that is organic and safe for my Nervous System. I would also invest in training for healthy food preparation, fitness, time management and organization. And, if I count my entire family's (myself, wife and child) health care costs totaling $21,000 per year, I am sure I can afford everything mentioned above *and* take my family on a yearly vacation.

I have worked with people that are considered to be among the wealthiest of the world, and powerful families wielding empires in business and generational wealth. In many cases, these individuals and families would trade everything they have to cure a sick, ailing or damaged loved one.

Health wisdom is free. A seed that grows into a plant that bears fruit accomplishes this simply by existing. The seed does not have to go to a seed school, or be trained in a seed specialty or become genetically modified and doused with synthetic chemicals to thrive. Our Nervous System knows the direction of healing as plants know the direction of the sun.

The bottom line is: all the riches of the world cannot help if you do not understand these five basic principles of Nervous System consciousness and healing. Focus all your resources toward developing your Nervous System. We are looking at stressful times ahead. Population issues, food availability with high prices for oil and transportation costs. You cannot eat your money, but you can use the money you have to feed and support your Nervous System.

Feeding your Nervous System obviously entails eating the best available foods. It also includes feeding your mind. Your Nervous System does not shut off; it is always "on." It thrives on being stimulated and expanded. As a child's curiosity expands his or her mind, we must endeavor to stimulate curiosity and conceptual conversation throughout our lives. Einstein claimed that he had no special talent, that he was only passionately curious.

You Have to Want It!

What is health worth to you? The government is not likely to hand over the control of how your health care dollars are spent. In my opinion, health is wealth! So, how do you afford to care for yourself? First and foremost, you have to want it! You have to demand it of yourself.

I ask you to commit to yourself and hold yourself accountable to the following. I will strive to:

- Honor and acknowledge myself in my Nervous System from this moment forward.

- Avoid anything that damages my Nervous System.

- Minimize the burden of synthetic chemicals on my Nervous System.

- Avoid genetically modified foods.

- Love myself for who I am and where I am in my life.

- Be of integrity and grow in all areas of my life.

- Do everything in my power to support the health of my Nervous System.

- Actively share the healing principles of the Nervous System with others.

Your holographic projection and your mind-set on health and healing contribute to the world's understanding of healing. In sharing these principles, you are actively choosing health that is sustainable for the world.

Learning does not stop when we leave school. We do not have to read a book to learn something new or to expand our Nervous System. When you make Nervous System cultivation and expansion the central focus of your life, you develop the most amazing Nervous System you can have. Within that target you will place your family, health, financial and spiritual dreams. We must remember that all our dreams are accomplished through our Nervous System. In focusing our attention, and cultivating the instrument that makes our dreams a reality, we can generate the reality of our wildest dreams.

I invite you to visit my website, where you can read more about and experience the healing of this work. It is my great honor to present it to you. When I developed this work, I had no idea that it would touch so many lives. Please tell your family, friends, doctors, neurologists and therapists about the power of Nervous System rehabilitation. I truly hope that Quantum Neurology® rehabilitation can be the answer for your needs.

For more information:
Contact the doctor nearest you

Review our Case Studies and Videos

Learning Quantum Neurology®
Seminars, Products & DVDs
www.QuantumNeurology.com

About the Author

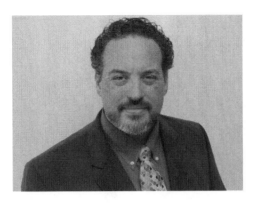

George Gonzalez, DC, QN
Chiropractor, Quantum Neurologist™

Dr. George Gonzalez is a renowned lecturer and expert in the activation and expansion of the Nervous System. He has developed a patented, systematic process for evaluating and correcting the Nervous System that began while researching a solution for his wife's spinal cord injury. The collection of techniques that led to her full recovery became Quantum Neurology® Rehabilitation. This advanced nerve rehabilitation system has provided countless patients improvement in their injury, illness or condition.

Dr. Gonzalez is the author of numerous articles, case studies and video trainings to support the development of Nervous System guided care. He has consulted with companies and has lectured to thousands of doctors worldwide. Additionally, he consults doctors who treat amateur and pro-athletes, chronically ill and disabled patients, autism spectrum disorders, stroke and brain injury repair, to name a few. He has lectured his revolutionary concepts internationally since early 2000.

Website: www.QuantumNeurology.com